POLICY
IS
PERSONAL

POLICY IS PERSONAL

Sex, gender, and informal care

CLARE UNGERSON

TAVISTOCK PUBLICATIONS

London and New York

First published in 1987 by
Tavistock Publications Ltd
11 New Fetter Lane, London
EC4P 4EE

Published in the USA by
Tavistock Publications
in association with Methuen, Inc.
29 West 35th Street, New York
NY 10001

© 1987 Clare Ungerson

Printed in Great Britain
by Richard Clay, Bungay, Suffolk

*British Library Cataloguing in
Publication Data*

Ungerson, Clare
Policy is personal: sex, gender and
informal care.
1. Aged—Home care—Great Britain
I. Title
649.8   HV1481.G5

ISBN 0–422–78500–8
ISBN 0–422–78510–5 Pbk

*Library of Congress Cataloging in
Publication Data*

Ungerson, Clare
Policy is personal.
"Published in the USA . . .
in association with
Methuen"—T.p. verso
Bibliography: p.
Includes index.
1. Aged—Home care—England—
Canterbury—Case studies.
2. Aged—England—Canterbury
—Family relationships—Case studies.
3. Aged—Intergenerational
relations—England—
Canterbury—Case studies.
I. Title
HV1481.G55C368 1987
362.6′092   87–10215

ISBN 0–422–78500–8
ISBN 0–422–78510–5 (pbk.)

To the memory of my grandmothers:

Lilli Jordan Gumbel
Dora Isbicki Ungerson

Contents

Acknowledgements

This book could not have been written without the kindness and consideration shown to me by the nineteen carers who welcomed me into their homes and told me about their lives. I am deeply grateful, and hope that the book that follows to some extent reflects their feelings as carers and their hopes for the book itself. David Oliviere, one time Principal Social Worker for Kent County Council, and instigator and guiding light of the Canterbury and Villages Carers' Support Group, was in at the inception of this research project and was tremendously generous with both his time and encouraging advice. The Economic and Social Research Council provided me with the grant that paid for the year's leave I took from teaching at the University of Kent; I am grateful to all my social policy and women's studies colleagues for rearranging their teaching so that I could take a year away.

As I have written this book, various people, some unknowingly, have considerably helped me with it. John Baldock, the late and deeply missed Joan Cartwright, Gill Davies, Mary Evans, Janet Sayers, and Julia Twigg either read the manuscript and commented very helpfully, or did or said something about caring which suddenly threw a whole new light on an issue.

Clare Ungerson,
University of Kent at Canterbury

1

Introduction: policy is personal

'Caring' is news. Both policies for community care and the position of informal carers in the home are regularly discussed in the serious press and on television. For example, in 1986 Neil Kinnock spoke of the position of informal carers in his rallying speech to the Labour Party Conference; Mrs Jacqueline Drake, who took a test case to the European Court of Justice claiming that married women should be able to claim the Invalid Care Allowance and won, became something of a household name; and the National Audit Commission reported on resources for community care and found them seriously wanting (1986). At the same time, the academic literature on caring, formal and informal, at home and in the neighbourhood, continued to grow apace. The literature on informal caring alone is now so large that bibliographical and research reviews have been found necessary, and two particularly useful reviews have recently been published (Parker 1985, Willmott 1986).

My reasons for adding to this literature are twofold. First, my interest in carers and the work that they do arises out of my own biography. The fact that my mother was a carer and looked after my grandmother in our home until my grandmother's death when I was 14 combines with the knowledge that, as an only daughter, my future contains the distinct possibility that I will sooner or later become a carer myself. As a result of the experience of living in a carer's household as a child, and because of the expectation that I too will become a carer, I am aware that there is a major gap in the burgeoning caring literature. The way particular carers in family constellations emerge, the way that carers talk about and construe the feelings they have about their work, the impact of caring on the relationship between carer and cared for: these are all issues that I know from experience to be important. Yet they are very little discussed in the literature – except in so far as it is possible to show that carers are under stress (Levin, Sinclair, and Gorbach 1983, Wright 1986). Stress and strain are certainly important feelings that a great many carers report, even to the extent of severe depressions and anxieties; but, again from my own experience, it seems to me that there are also far more complicated and contradictory feelings at work. Most of this book is concerned with a discussion of these complications.

The second set of reasons for writing this book is that it accords with and is fed by my own commitment to woman-centred issues and to feminism. It has almost reached the dimensions of banality to claim that most carers are women; nevertheless, given the accuracy of that statement, it seems to me necessary to explore the full implications of the fact. If most carers are women, do women carers feel that what they do is particularly compatible with their female identity? Do men carers feel emasculated? How do women carers feel about caring for men? How do men carers feel about caring for women? There is more to a feminist approach to knowledge than the documentation of the role of women in a set of social processes; while this is important, it is also necessary (and even exciting) to use issues of sex and gender to illuminate those very social processes. The topics discussed in this book are always considered from a gendered perspective; in other words, I have tried throughout to think about the issues by asking the question, do sex and gender make a difference? (The answer, of course, is that they almost always do.)

This study of nineteen people, who, in 1984, were looking after someone elderly and frail, has a long and instructive history. My initial interest in carers arose out of my participation in the women's movement in the early 1970s. When I looked at my own life it seemed obvious that there were elements in it that had profoundly shaped it and the life of the woman (my mother), but not that of the man (my father), with whom I had shared much of that life. These elements were going to continue to shape my life in a way that they would shape no man's. My mother had been a 'carer' of her own mother throughout my childhood; as an only daughter it never occurred to me (and still does not) that there were alternatives when I thought about the care of my parents in their old age. Apart from a vague notion of some form of public-sector care (my other grandmother had lived her last seven years in the back ward of a depressing mental hospital in south-east London), I knew that my mother's example was the one I would have to follow, however restrictive it had proved to be in her life or disruptive it would be of mine. For the first time in my life I came to understand how the state and social policy, which I studied in my academic work in their effects on the poor and disadvantaged, were inevitably going to have an enormous impact on me personally. Despite being, through my paid work, relatively affluent and well endowed with occupational pensions, unmarried and hence not regulated by family law, without children and so unlikely to have to negotiate the schools system, I suddenly realized, at the age of 26 and with fit and healthy parents, that state policies for the care of the elderly were of immense, continuing and direct interest to me.

At the same time, alternating Labour and Conservative governments were developing a consensus about the future of state provision of care for the elderly. These are the policies, begun in the late 1950s with the 1959 Mental Health Act and continued into the 1960s and 1970s with various plans and policy documents (for a history of these plans, see Henwood 1986), now known generally as policies for 'community care'. As a student in the mid-1960s I had read a great deal of criticism of these policies, directed largely at the lack of co-ordination between on the one hand, the hospital boards, which were planning to reduce the number of hospital beds, and, on the other hand, the local authorities which would be largely responsible for providing support services in 'the community' (*A Hospital Plan for England and Wales*, 1962; *Health and Welfare: The Development of Community Care*, 1963). This lack of co-ordination was usually presented as a difficulty that could be resolved administratively through better planning, and as yet another indication of how the so-called 'tripartite' National Health Service failed to operate efficiently and sensibly. The issue of what, in reality, constituted 'community care', and even what might constitute it if ever there were adequate co-ordination between the two bureaucracies of health and welfare, was largely left untouched.

There were only two commentators who seemed to me to bring the issue alive and closer to home: Peter Townsend, in his study of old people living at home and in institutions (1957, 1962), and Richard Titmuss, in his essay on 'Community Care: Fact or Fiction' (first published in 1963, later republished in his book of essays, *Commitment to Welfare*, 1968). As a student, I read Peter Townsend's beautifully written *The Family Life of Old People* (1957) from cover to cover without putting it down. The focus of the book was on the lives and family structure of 203 elderly men and women living in the old London borough of Bethnal Green. Townsend himself interviewed the majority of the respondents; his lively and loving descriptions of the old Bethnal Green 'characters' leapt off every page, and there were travel-writer style descriptions of the 'colour' of Bethnal Green street life. At the same time aspects of the lives of the old people were carefully quantified: their family structures (some of them enormous), their contact with close kin, their incomes, and their recent state of health. The essential argument of the book was that Bethnal Green was a matriarchal society where reciprocal caring was carried out by women, vertically between the generations and horizontally between kin, with the grandmother at the apex:

> 'Men, young as well as old, rarely occupied a vital role in family care. The system was chiefly organised around female relatives. At its focal point stood the old woman ... she usually retained important functions as housewife, mother and grandmother. ... Usually she managed the home, be it with increasing assistance from her daughters and other relatives ... it is hardly possible to over-emphasise the way in which the old women, even when infirm, continued to occupy an important place in the family.'
>
> (Townsend 1957:53–4)

'For the majority of women increasing age was a gradual unwinding of the springs of life. They gave up part-time occupations, visits to the cinema, shopping, cleaning and washing, services for neighbours and associations with them, friendships outside the family, holidays and week-ends with relatives, the care of the grandchildren, the provision of meals for children, and finally their own cooking and budgeting, one by one as their faculties grew dim and age took its toll. Their last refuge was their family. They did not want to escape from their homes, to a cottage in the country any more than to an institution. They wanted to spend their last months in their homes and among their families, where possessions and faces were familiar and where an unsteady foot was most secure.

'Their activities became adjusted to a limited routine. They went out little and slept longer. They bemoaned their frailty but even when wholly incapacitated they kept, because they were women and not men it was said, "a closer touch on things". They knew what was happening to their relatives, had a finger on the details of family history, and were respected and admired for their canniness and insight into what went on. "She's a marvel, really", said more than one daughter, "she's got such spirit and she can still have a laugh."'

(Townsend 1957: 55–6)

Despite the power and attractiveness of Townsend's writing, the vividness with which he depicted the life of Bethnal Green, the fact that he took sex and gender into account at every point, the book nevertheless seemed at the time to bear little relation to the kind of family life of old people with which I was personally familiar. He was describing a system of solidarity that was stable, unitary, and based on kinship and locality. There was little or no mention of the position of those old people whose family networks had been geographically or socially mobile. In other words, the relationships described in the book depended on a certain insularity, consolidated by the solidarity bred by employment in the docks and the continuity of a working-class life-style founded on extensive kinship networks and large families still based in a particular locality. This seemed a long way from my own experience of middle-class life, with a small family, widely dispersed.

Even in the mid-1960s the Townsend book (1957) was beginning to take on the characteristics of a historical document. It was scarcely credible that the life he had described less than ten years earlier could survive the closure of the docks, the out-migration of many of the younger families, and the immigration of numbers of Asians to the area. Clearly, even Bethnal Green could change – and, indeed, in a recent study has been shown to have done so radically (Holme 1985). Further, given Townsend's interpretation of Bethnal Green family life as largely matriarchal and gerontocratic, and the system of caring as reciprocal, he seemed to suggest that carers, almost all of whom he acknowledged to be women, were powerful and prestigious *because they were carers*. Once again, this ran contrary to my experience. In my own small family, caring had not seemed to carry power or prestige; on the contrary, the caring relationships I had observed in my childhood had seemed difficult precisely because carer and cared for had each felt power*less*. Far from generating prestige, the inherent privacy of the caring relationship removed it from the public eye and hence, in a small family, from public approbation.

Thus Townsend's book was both fascinating and disappointing. For the first time, the reality of care was spelled out – in terms of shopping and cooking, cleaning and washing. Yet, at the same time, the cheerfulness with which that care was carried out and the multiple carers selected and rewarded seemed totally remote from my experience. Moreover, the seductive descriptions of powerful old matriarchs, respected and cared for by their grateful female kin in the bosom of their families, made it all too easy to slip from realism to idealism, from what is to what ought to be. Even before the onslaught of feminism, I felt distinctly uncomfortable.

The other major work on community care which I read as a student and which spoke more closely to my own experience was that of Richard Titmuss. In his essay 'Community Care: Fact or Fiction?' (1968), Titmuss did not refer at all to informal carers or to women. But the power of this short essay lay in his ironic treatment of the term 'community care':

'What some hope will one day exist is suddenly thought by many to exist already. All kinds of wild and unlovely weeds are changed, by statutory magic and comforting appellation, into the most attractive flowers that bloom not just in the spring but all the year round. We are all familiar with that exotic hot-house climbing rose, "The Welfare State", with its lovely hues of tender pink and blushing red, rampant and rampaging all over the place, often preventing people from "standing on their own feet" in their own gardens. And what of the everlasting cottage-garden trailer, "Community Care"? Does it not conjure up a sense of warmth and human kindness, essentially personal and comforting, as loving as the wild flowers so enchantingly described by Lawrence in *Lady Chatterley's Lover*?'

(Titmuss 1968: 104)

It was not just Titmuss's juxtaposition of wishful thinking with reality that made me smile with recognition, it was also the dissonance between his description of the loving kindness which the word 'care', in this context, was intended to mean, and the reality of difficulty that I knew it could create.

During the decade of the 1960s another strand of work developed, relevant to the issue of informal care, concerning the effects on residents of long-term institutional care. Peter Townsend's own study of *The Last Refuge: A Survey of Residential Institutions and Homes of Old People* (1962) was the first of many British studies documenting the insensitivity and even brutality that appeared to prevail within a variety of institutional settings. (These *Ideas on Institutions* have since been reviewed in a highly critical but useful manner by Kathleen Jones and A. J. Fowles (1984).) Such studies formed part of the growing chorus of disapproval for residential care; and they provided the intellectual and moral basis for the political consensus concerning the alternative of care in and by 'the community' (Henwood 1986). These critiques held some personal meaning for me; my father's mother was at the time suffering from senile dementia and a resident in a long-term geriatric ward in a large mental hospital. Without speech or personality, with none of her belongings around her, wearing communal clothes and clumsily cut hair, this thin and toothless person known as 'Mrs Ungerson' seemed to be neither my grandmother nor my grandfather's wife. Yet, on my occasional visits to her in the company of my grandfather, who visited her daily, I knew that she seemed well cared for. I also recognized that the act of seeing her every day and helping her with her lunch gave my elderly grandfather a much needed structure to his day, as well as the regular pleasure of recognition and respect from the welcoming nurses. There were clearly gains as well as losses in such a formal and institutional system of care.

Towards the end of the 1960s and into the early 1970s some research attention shifted back to care in the community. Probably the most important work to emerge during this period was Michael Bayley's study of informal caring (1973). In that book he described the lives of a small number of families caring for their mentally subnormal adult children; his graphic phrase 'the daily grind', used to describe the day-to-day routine of those families, has now moved into the vernacular of the general caring literature. What impressed me, and others, about that book, apart from its documentary realism, was the fact that almost all the caring work, including carrying fully grown handicapped adults up and down stairs, was carried out by the mothers in the families. Fathers 'helped'; mothers bore the brunt – always with stoicism, often with dedication and love. Of course this was not news; woman-centred caring was precisely what Townsend had described in Bethnal Green. What was new was the description of caring stripped of any nostalgia or romanticism. Caring was, as Bayley described it, literally onerous, emotionally demanding, hardly reciprocal, and only rarely rewarding.

At about this moment, in the mid-1970s, the first stirrings of a feminist critique of policies for community care began to filter through. In common with other feminist teachers of social administration I used Michael Bayley's book in my standard teaching, alongside Titmuss's essay, to argue that there was a hidden agenda for women within such policies. In 1976 a thoughtful but implicitly extremely anti-feminist book – R. M. Moroney's *The Family and the State: Considerations for Social Policy* (1976) – added fuel to the tiny fire. This short book, published in the USA as well as in Britain and reprinted in 1978, was, and still is, widely quoted. While providing a wealth of useful data on trends in need and provision for the elderly and the mentally handicapped over the past century, the book also made the unquestioning assumption that carers were women and that carers should be women. Moroney referred throughout to 'family care' and never to 'woman care'; yet, in probably the most significant section of the book, he classified women as the 'caretaker pool':

'The caretaker ratio developed in Table 2.5 is built on two potential sources of care: married and single women between the ages of forty-five and sixty. In 1901, for every 100 elderly persons in the general population, there were eighty-three women aged forty-five to fifty-nine, of whom thirteen were single, almost a one to one ratio. Fifty years later this ratio had dropped sharply and by 1971 it had been halved. While the number of women forty-five to sixty had increased from 6 to 8 per cent (keeping in mind that the majority are working) the number of elderly grew from less than 8 to 19 per cent. Shifts among single women in this age group are even more strik-ing. Whereas there were thirteen spinsters (1901) for every 100 elderly, now there are only five. Shifts in marital status have been sharp since the war. Approximately 14 per cent of all women between forty-five and sixty were unmarried in 1901. By 1971 only 8 per cent were unmarried. The caretaker pool has been effectively reduced by demographic changes (shifts in age structure and marital status) and competing demands on time.'

(Moroney 1976: 22)

The major new problem identified by Moroney was that, now and for the predictable future, there simply would not be enough women to go round – particularly women whose energies were not distracted by husbands and/or paid work. Such full-blooded sexism in an otherwise thoughtful book was a some-what ambiguous teaching tool. Nevertheless, given the scarcity of a feminist critique of community care policies in the mid-1970s, Moroney's work could be, and was, a useful way of focusing students' minds on the sexist assumptions underlying contemporary commentary.

By the end of the 1970s a small feminist literature concerning community care began to emerge. Articles by Hilary Land (Who Cares for the Family?, 1978) and, a year later, Mary McIntosh (The Welfare State and the Needs of the Dependent Family, 1979) presaged a small onrush of other work critical of govern-ment policy for community care in respect of its impact on women. In the same year David Wilkin (1979) published a book describing in some detail the sexual division of labour in house-holds caring for mentally handicapped children. But the water-shed came with a paper by Janet Finch and Dulcie Groves, given first at a Social Administration Association conference in the summer of 1979, and then published by them in the *Journal of Social Policy* the following year. In 'Community Care and the Family: A Case for Equal Opportunities?' (1980) they argued that policies for community care were, within a context of public expenditure cuts, fundamentally incompatible with policies for equal opportunity for women. Echoing Moroney's unconscious solecism, Finch and Groves spelt out what they called a 'double equation': 'that in practice community care equals care by the family, and in practice care by the family equals care by women' (p. 494). A month after the publication of their article, in November 1980, Janet Finch and Dulcie Groves held a very small conference at the University of Lancaster on 'Women, Work and Caring' the papers for which, along with others, were later published in their important and much cited book *A Labour of Love: Women, Work and Caring* (1983). The organization of feminist academics around the issue of community care had begun with a flourish.

In the late 1970s research funding bodies had begun to support studies of the position of women as carers. Prominent among them was the Equal Opportunities Commission (EOC), which in 1977 had commissioned a study of carers from a survey research firm. The first problem, as in all succeeding surveys, was to find some carers. A postal survey of 2,500 households in West Yorkshire, with a response rate of only 36 per cent, gave rise to 116 interviews with carers. For the first time a serious effort had been made to plot the incidence of caring and to discover the sex ratio. Out of the 116 carers, 87 (75 per cent) were women and 29 (25 per cent) were men. The survey was significant not only for its quantitative elements (which, given the low response to the initial postal survey, had to be treated with considerable caution); it also documented, through the medium of lengthy quotes from the 116 in-depth interviews, the considerable emotional and financial stress with which carers struggled (EOC 1980). As a result of this survey, the EOC moved into the forefront of the critique of government policy. In 1982 it published a research report summarizing the chief findings to date about women and caring (EOC 1982a), and a set of recommendations for the support of carers, in terms of services, financial benefits, and employment rights (1982b). For a government-funded body, the EOC proved to be much more than a paper tiger when it came to a critique of government policy. For example (and there are many similar statements to choose from in this document):

> 'The carers visible to Government statisticians are married men aged less than 65 years old caring for their disabled wives, and single people caring for infirm parents. Carers are only visible to policy-makers when they receive some kind of state benefit, yet many welfare benefits exclude married women. ... The official invisibility of carers contributes to their disadvantage by allowing policy-makers to ignore the consequences of care by the community.'
>
> (EOC 1982b:3)

Other funding bodies also took up the issue. In 1980 the Joseph Rowntree Memorial Trust – which had earlier supported Moroney's (1976) research – funded, in conjunction with the Equal Opportunities Commission, Muriel Nissel and Lucy Bonnerjea's work at the Policy Studies Institute. The purpose of their study was to 'examine the extent to which the caring functions of the family operate as a constraint on women's participation in the community on an equal footing with men' (Nissel and Bonnerjea 1982:4). What emerged, largely as a result of the brilliant device of using time diaries, was that, in a sample of forty-four married-couple households caring for an elderly dependent relative, the wives spent on average between two and three hours every day undertaking essential care for the relative – irrespective of whether the wives were in paid employment or not – and the husbands spent *eight minutes*! When Nissel and Bonnerjea came to cost the time spent by women carers on all aspects of caring they concluded that, using the market rates for home helps and other domestic helpers prevailing in 1980, these women were doing work that would, under different and paid circumstances, generate an income of £47.50 a week. If the earnings forgone by women who had given up work in order to care were also taken into account, then these women were also losing, on average, a further £87.00 per week. Clearly the government was getting a very good deal!

Finally, the government-funded Social Science Research Council (SSRC) also entered the fray. In 1980 the Sociology and Social Administration Committee of the SSRC (now renamed

the Economic and Social Research Council) launched two research initiatives, one of which was on the 'caring capacity of
the community'. In its circular letter inviting academics to bid
for the small amount of funding that was available, the committee mentioned feasibility projects designed to explore, first, the
relationship between formal and informal sources of care and,
second, the relationship between providers and users of formal
and informal help (SSRC 1980). At the very end of the letter
reference was made to the possibility of funding a 'research
review' into 'the impact of the growing numbers of women
entering the labour market' on the caring capacity of the
community.

My personal response to this letter was a great deal of heart-
searching. The opportunity to speculate about the relationship
between structural factors such as the labour market, the position
of women generally, and the policy of community care seemed
too good to be passed over. Yet it was obvious that two distinct
schools of thought had emerged; one view saw government
policy as the 'problem', particularly for women; the other saw
demographic and social change, particularly the growth in the
numbers of the elderly, the reduction of family size, and the
increasing use of women's time in the paid labour market, as the
'problem'. The request for the research review was the only
aspect of the SSRC initiative that seemed to take account of the
sexed and gendered nature of the 'caring capacity of the community'. Yet the way the request was phrased seemed to indicate a view of women which, by implication, referred back to
Moroney's entirely female 'caretaker pool'. Eventually I decided
that, given the context of a 'research review', it might be possible to suggest research questions which, rather than confirm
the apparent reduction of the 'caretaker pool' as a problem in
itself, could build on and develop further the feminist perspective on community care that was being developed so rapidly
elsewhere. In 1980, in a proposal which made it quite clear
which side of the fence I was on, I applied for, and (somewhat to
my surprise) obtained, the SSRC grant necessary to give me
time off teaching in order to apply myself full-time to the needs
of the research review.

The issue concerning the future of the 'caring capacity of the
community' and the expanding participation of women in the

labour market seemed to me fairly easy to tackle within a single over-arching hypothesis. Given the strength of the ideology of women as nurturers, and the economics of the labour market and women's subordinate position within it, it seemed extremely unlikely that women would, in the foreseeable future, overturn their traditional position as society's carers. I argued that women's entry into the labour market had been characterized by their entry into work on a part-time basis and that there was plenty of evidence, drawn from labour market economics and from attitudinal surveys, that women's behaviour in the labour market was dominated by their perception of their family's needs rather more than by any other personal or pecuniary motivation. The researchable issues I proposed were, in general, designed to test the hypothesis that even if other parts of women's lives, particularly their participation in paid work, had apparently changed very considerably, the position of women as carers was likely to change very little. There were, however, some possible changes which I thought *might* alter women's perception of themselves as primarily mothers and nurturers: the possibility, particularly in some labour markets, that women's employment would remain more buoyant than men's, thus perhaps leading to some role-swapping within households; the possibility that relativities in the labour market between men's and women's earning potential would become more equal, such that the differential opportunity costs of men and women stopping work in order to care for someone were drastically reduced; the possibility that the increasing incongruence of the assumptions of much Welfare State legislation, particularly in the field of social security, with women's growing participation in the labour market would lead to some attitudinal change on the part of women, and women's increasing political activity in protest at their treatment in the labour market and by the welfare organs of the state. While suggesting all these as interesting research issues, I was also in my own mind fairly confident that none of these changes would take place, let alone have any or much impact on women's traditional caring role. (This part of the research review was later published as 'Why Do Women Care' (Ungerson 1983a) in Janet Finch and Dulcie Groves's book, *A Labour of Love: Women, Work and Caring*, 1983, previously mentioned; the second part of the review was later published in a collection of papers given at the 1982 annual conference of the British Sociological Association (Ungerson 1983b).)

The second part of the research review seemed to me to be more interesting because it was the more speculative part of the task I had set for myself. Given that women were going to continue, as I had argued in the first part of the review, to predominate among carers, I wanted to know what implications this fact, in itself, might have on the relationship between carers and cared for. I was also interested in speculating how far issues of sex and gender of carer and cared for might have a generalizable impact on the quality of the caring relationship. There seemed very little, if any, relevant literature concerned with these issues, and I came to realize that the only way I could begin to think about them was to consider how I myself might feel as a woman carer. This ran contrary to my previous social-scientific training, where personal experience was, if possible, to be excluded from rational and intellectual exercise. However, it seemed that such elevation of personal experience and feelings to the realms of intellectual endeavour had been given legitimacy by the women's movement through its statement that 'the personal is political'. At the time I was thinking about the research review, the sociologist Margaret Stacey, then president of the British Sociological Association, was herself advocating in a widely circulated and later published paper that

> 'We must admit the importance of feeling states over a wider range than the recognition of consciousness of the kind which we are familiar with in class formation . . . it has been a major contribution of the recent women's movement to put feelings, experiences, consciousness on the agenda for political action; to insist that politics cannot be understood without taking account of the politics of the family, of the experiences of women in their relationships with men . . . a similar point has to be made with regard to sociological theory.'
>
> (Stacey 1981:189)

I felt I had been 'given permission' to go ahead and lean on my own psyche as the generator of research ideas.

The focus of my attention was on the relationship between carer and cared for, and how far it could be argued that sex and

gender determined the nature and quality of that caring relationship. By looking hard into my own experience and feelings,
I eventually came up with four issues which I thought were
particularly important:

(1) The historical biography of the relationship between carer
    and cared for: how far was it possible for people with a long
    history on one particular basis to continue to relate to each
    other on the level of physical intimacy, laced with disgust,
    that caring often demands? Given that many of these long-
    standing relationships will have been based on generally
    agreed and understood norms of behaviour (e.g. parents
    and children, husbands and wives), were there particular
    difficulties of adjustment to the new caring situation – for
    example, where carer and cared for were married to each
    other? How easy was it for children to become quasi-parents,
    and in particular were there special difficulties of shifting
    power relations between mothers and daughters?

(2) Were there similarities between caring and mothering, such
    that, particularly where carers were women, carers con-
    structed their tasks as mothering and infantilized the people
    they were caring for?

(3) Were there particular problems about disgust with bodily
    functions no longer under 'proper' control and sex-related
    taboos about them, such that men – even willing ones –
    withdrew from the management of incontinence, leaving
    that management to women as their more 'proper' sphere,
    thus re-confirming the predominant sexual division of
    labour in caring?

(4) Finally, were there particular problems about what I called
    'cross-sex caring' between kin – i.e. men and women caring
    for blood-related kin of the opposite sex – such that the
    operation of the incest taboos created particular difficulties?
    (Since I wrote, in 1980, about the possible impact of incest
    taboos on the caring relationship, there has been growing
    public concern about the widespread nature of incestuous
    practice and its long-standing and enormous impact on a
    whole range of human relationships; e.g. Renvoize 1982. No
    doubt the operation of an informal caring relationship be-
    tween one-time incestuous partners, particularly fathers and
    daughters, would be well nigh impossible.)

Given the intimacy of the issues I had outlined, it was clear that, in order to research them, only qualitative methods would do. Such qualitative research would in itself be extremely difficult. For example, how does one ask people about taboo in a way that does not transgress the taboo itself? My final suggestion to the SSRC committee was that small-scale feasibility studies should be funded to discover how far it was possible to ask such questions within the context of a short-term study (Ungerson 1981). In the event, in 1983 I applied to the SSRC to do such a study myself. The issue as to how far one can begin to discover the operation of taboos, and more specifically their impact on the caring relationship, remains unresolved. But the book that follows is the end-product of that research process; it is rooted in the women's movement and my own biography, and watered and fed by feminist academic friends and colleagues, and, last but not least, by the Economic and Social Research Council.

2
The sample survey: its methodology and the respondents

This research project was carried out in 1984 and is based on what until fairly recently would have been regarded as an absurdly and illegitimately small sample. It was always intended that this survey of carers should be on a very small scale and that its results would be highly qualitative and interpretative. In my original research proposal I suggested that no more than twenty carers should be interviewed, and there were in fact nineteen respondents. The reason for keeping the sample to such small numbers was that the chief original purpose of the survey was to explore the emotional context of caring and in particular to discover whether my ideas about the impact of certain taboos, namely those concerning incest and the management of human incontinence, would have any differential effect on how the two sexes felt about caring (see Chapter 1). It seemed to me that what was needed was an exploratory, open-ended interview schedule whose main purpose would be to establish whether or not examination of these 'taboo topics' was feasible in the context of one or two meetings with a few carers. Thus the intention of the survey was, from the outset, strictly qualitative; I wanted carers to talk intimately to me about intimate issues. Issues that could be quantified – for example, the time and financial costs of caring, and its morale costs – seemed to me to have been more than adequately tackled by other excellent research work (see, for example, Nissel and Bonnerjea 1982, Baldwin 1985, Levin, Sinclair and Gorbach 1983).

In the event the particular questions that I had designed to elicit and elucidate these 'taboo topics' did not work very well, and in this book answers to these questions are referred to only where they shed some light on other issues. Part of the problem with these particular questions is that I left them to the end of the questionnaire, assuming that by then I might have developed some intimate rapport with the carer, who would then be prepared to articulate taboo feelings. However, the interviews unexpectedly turned out to be very long (usually about two hours, and many of the respondents were seen twice for up to two hours at a time); this meant that by the time I reached these questions both the carer and myself were often exhausted. With some of the respondents it seemed counter-productive to ask the questions at all, and on these occasions I abandoned them altogether. Moreover, many of the respondents who did answer these questions gave answers based on their personal knowledge of carers in a particular kin relationship with the person they were caring for, claiming that they could not answer for caring relationships of which they themselves had no experience or close knowledge. A typical response to a question asking if they thought there were any 'problems' about a son caring for his mother was, 'I'm not sure. I don't know anyone in that situation'. (See Ungerson 1985a for a fuller discussion of the difficulties that arose about these particular questions and my conclusion that one would do better to interview a sample from the general population rather than carers only.)

Thus, in one major respect, the reason for aiming for a very small sample had to fall by the wayside. Nevertheless, it seems to me that many of the other issues that arose in the course of the interviews, particularly about personal biography between carer and cared for and its impact on feelings about their caring relationship, and the differences in the way men and women talked about and constructed their role as carers, could have emerged only with in-depth interviews conducted by the same interviewer. I was also convinced by the literature on what constitutes 'feminist research' and its burgeoning product (Roberts 1981) that there were enormous benefits in in-depth and open-ended interviews if they were carried out by the same interviewer and so that the respondents could themselves partly determine how and where the research went. Such a two-way process between researcher and researched would be far more difficult, if not impossible, with a large sample entailing pre-coded questions and a great deal of computing and eventual statistical analysis. But this book is not about how to conduct social research, let alone 'feminist' research. It seems to me that the proof of the pudding can lie only in the eating; so, after this somewhat perfunctory explanation of the sample size, I turn to the sample itself.

THE SAMPLING FRAME

Carers are notoriously difficult to find. It is the nature of informal caring that it is done behind closed doors. Given lack of information or an unfounded certainty that the social services would not be available for the likes of them, it can safely be assumed that large numbers of carers never bring themselves to the attention of their local Social Services Department (SSD) or even make their domestic responsibilities clear to their general practitioner (GP). In this particular study I was fortunate to live and work in a local-authority area where carers were taken very seriously by the SSD, and where one local social worker in particular had taken it upon himself to help organize a Carers' Support Group in Canterbury and the surrounding villages. I was fortunate to gain access to members of the Carers' Support Group via the SSD.

The people interviewed were contacted through a list of 'carers' kept by the local SSD. This list is supposed to contain the names of all those who have, within the last two or three years, been in contact with the SSD and made it clear that their reason for getting in touch is because they are caring for someone elderly, whether as a neighbour or a relative, whether living in the same dwelling as the elderly person or living near by. As far as the SSD is concerned this list has one overriding purpose: to build up a mailing list of people to whom a newsletter on caring is regularly sent and to provide the nucleus of a Carers' Support Group to which a number of activities, such as courses for carers, guest speakers at large meetings, and a 'sitter service', are attached. Thus this list is not service based or client based in

any systematic way. In other words, it is not possible to generalize either about the nature of the service that people on the
list are receiving or about the extent or nature of the dependency
of the elderly person for whom they are apparently caring. It
is even impossible to assume that the term 'elderly' can be
applied to all the people who are being cared for by the carers
on this mailing list, since the ages of the cared for are not
systematically recorded; however, because the Carers' Support
Group was at the time of the interviews run by the Principal
Social Worker specializing in the care of the elderly, the list does
definitely exclude those caring for the relatively young and
middle-aged.

Thus there are some people on this list whose only personal
contact with the SSD has been a telephone enquiry about the
provision of a particular service and who, in the course of that
call, were told that the service was not available or that they
were not eligible for it. In contrast, there are others on the list
who are well known to the department and in receipt of a large
number of services, including day care for the person they are
caring for, home help, district nurse help, and attendance allowance. Some people on the mailing list are active participants in
the Support Group, attending meetings regularly and contributing to the newsletter. Others are totally passive 'members'
of the group whose only contact with it is their receipt of the
twice-yearly newsletter.

In short, there are very few generalizations that can be made
about the carers in this sampling frame. It is neither absolutely
clear how they came to be on the list in the first place, nor
possible to generalize about the nature of dependency of the
people they are caring for. Among the nineteen carers eventually interviewed, the people they were caring for featured a
wide variety of types of dependency. Some respondents were
looking after people with long histories of mental illness or
mental handicap; others were dealing with the very different
stages of senile dementia; yet others were looking after someone
with no mental incapacity whatever but who, through the con-
traction of an infectious illness at an early age, was highly
dependent physically or, as the result of a stroke, had lost the
power of speech but not the power of expression. One carer
denied that there was anything at all wrong with her mother-in-

law, but nevertheless fully understood the term, and recognized herself to be, a 'carer'.

In many ways the list of carers was itself an institutionalized form of all the difficulties and ambiguities surrounding the definition of 'caring'. In particular, because the Support Group was administered through the SSD, the meaning of the word 'caring' had taken on a bureaucratic and professional tone, stressing the tasks of caring *for* a person rather than the feelings of caring *about* one. As one of the people interviewed put it (almost as soon as I'd walked through her front door), 'I'm a *daughter*, not a carer!'. Even specialists giving lectures at the carers' course sometimes had the mistaken belief that they were addressing volunteer 'sitters' rather than informal carers. Some people were on the list because they had been referred from another agency such as a GP, but once identified as a 'carer' objected to that definition of themselves precisely because of its use within a bureaucratic rather than affective framework and because of the word's apparently distancing and occupational tone. Others were on the list because they had at some point decided that they should take responsibility for someone else's needs, if only to the minimal extent of finding out what the SSD might provide by way of assistance. They had thus put themselves forward as 'carers', but there was no way of knowing to what extent they were involved with the dependent elderly person unless the SSD, as a result of the 'carer's' initial enquiry, had developed a continuous relationship with the cared for. At the interview stage it became clear that for some of these people it was a source of pride to be recognized as a carer, and they regarded the description as wholly appropriate to their tasks and feelings; others felt uncomfortable to be identified in such a quasi-occupational way.

THE SAMPLE

All the people on the SSD carers' mailing list were initially written to by the Principal Social Worker who at that time ran the Carers' Support Group. A stamped addressed envelope was enclosed with the letter, and people were given approximately two weeks to reply. Of the 130 people initially contacted, 56 replied, of whom 32 said they were willing to participate in the study. Of these, 21 were resident within Canterbury, and I decided to restrict the sample to these Canterbury residents in order to avoid the further complicating factor of interviewing people in somewhat isolated villages or run-down seaside resorts. Efforts to interview all 21 Canterbury residents were made, but only 19 respondents were eventually interviewed, since one carer proved impossible to contact and another willingly made appointments but was out when I called at all three appointed times.

It is therefore not possible to make claims that, in social or demographic terms, this sample is particularly representative of anything. As has already been pointed out, the sampling frame itself contained a very wide variety of social and caring circumstances and an unplumbed and unanalysed collection of meanings. The fact that more than half the possible respondents declined to take part means that the remaining willing participants must be regarded as a somewhat self-selected group. As a result of the SSD's desire to maintain strict confidentiality it is not possible to say anything about those carers who declined to take part. However, during the interviews with the willing participants it often became clear why these particular respondents had put themselves forward for interview. Almost all of them had reached some kind of crisis point which they wanted to chew over, even with a totally unknown social researcher. For example, some – particularly the women respondents caring for an in-law – were worried about their own parents who were becoming increasingly frail. Others were reaching the end of their tether and wanted a space in which they could talk over the possibility of getting permanent residential care. Others had themselves become ill and were having physical difficulties with coping, while yet others were having to move house or, as a result of other members of their family moving house, were losing their immediate source of support. (These particular difficulties are discussed in context and detail in Chapters 5 and 6.) There were also reasons for wanting to participate which were less to do with the immediate circumstances and more with how they perceived themselves. For example, a number of the respondents were active members of the Carers' Support Group, to the extent of being on the organizing committee and regular attenders at meetings. Participation in a study of caring was, presumably, one more way of capturing the term and status of 'carer' for themselves. Others had a strong connection with higher education and were interested in contributing to knowledge or, at least, in finding out how someone went about 'doing' social research. Almost inevitably in a small town, one or two had very close connections with my own university, and others knew of me through personal friends who are my colleagues. All of the respondents had an enormous amount to say to me, and the interviews often spread over two visits, each of approximately two hours.

THE RESPONDENTS

In order to make it easier for the reader to place the analysis of the following chapters in its real-life context, in the following paragraphs I present a series of thumb-nail sketches of the people interviewed. All the names have been changed, and some details omitted, in order to preserve confidentiality.

The women carers

Mrs Archer *is in her middle fifties and works full-time as a clerical officer. She was born and bought up in Canterbury; both her children have left home. Both her parents are 79 years old and, having lived in very bad privately rented accommodation all their lives, have recently moved into a tiny but well-maintained almshouse. The Prioress keeps an eye out for them. Both Mrs Archer's parents are ill. Her father is showing the early signs of senile dementia, and her mother has Parkinson's disease and is seriously underweight. Her mother recently spent eight weeks in the local geriatric hospital to get her weight up and for observation. Mrs Archer visits her parents three times a week, and her father spends all Sunday with her and her husband. Mrs Archer does all her parents' housework and takes her mother out in her wheelchair. A district nurse washes her mother once a week.*

Mrs Barnes *is in her middle forties and cares for her mother-in-law. On marriage she gave up work as a nurse and has not had a paid job since. Two of her three children are at school and live at home. Her mother-in-law is 81 years old and has been ill with senile dementia for seven years. At the time of the first interview the old lady was in the* local general hospital, where she had been admitted for observation as a result of a number of falls and loss of appetite. By the time I interviewed Mrs Barnes for the second time the old lady had been moved to the local mental hospital for assessment but she was likely to be discharged at any time. Mrs Barnes's mother-in-law did not actually live with them; her house was in the same grounds as Mrs Barnes's house and within less than fifty yards' walk along a garden path. The two houses were within sight of one another. Due to her mother-in-law's propensity to wander, Mrs Barnes very reluctantly locked her in her house overnight. Understandably, Mrs Barnes was very worried about the possibility of a fire from which her mother-in-law could not escape. As a result of the crisis in her mother-in-law's life (described by Mrs Barnes as 'the crunch has come') the entire family was moving, the family estate being sold, and the old lady was going to move into a 'granny annexe' in the new house.

Mrs Cook is fifty and works every morning in the matron's office of a local boarding-school. Her son is at university and comes home during the vacations. Mrs Cook cares for her father, aged 85, who lives in a village some way out of Canterbury but on a railway line with a direct train service from Canterbury. Mrs Cook also cares for her aunt, who lives within easy walking distance. Her aunt is 72, and her aunt's husband is still alive; after various illnesses the aunt has been diagnosed as having cancer and is finding it increasingly difficult to move about. Mrs Cook's father is fit but old, and just before the interview had returned home after spending six weeks in Mr and Mrs Cook's home recovering from pleurisy. Mrs Cook is trying to discover ways in which the local authority might rehouse her father nearer to her own home. In order to make time to care for two elderly people, Mrs Cook gets up at 5 a.m., does her housework and gets to work at 7.40 a.m. At 12.30 p.m. she leaves work and catches a train to her father's, where she gives him his lunch and does his housework and shopping. At 3 p.m. she catches a train back to Canterbury and from 3.30 to 4.30 p.m. she does her aunt's housework and shopping. At 4.30 p.m. she returns home and gets her husband's tea. In the evening she does the ironing and washing for her own and the other two households. Mrs Cook's only contact with the Social Services Department has been to ask whether it could help pay for the installation of a telephone for her father. The SSD was unable to help.

Mrs Davies is 47 and cares for her father-in-law, who is 77. Mrs Davies works three full days a week at the local general hospital. Twelve *years ago, on the death of his wife, her father-in-law moved from Scotland and took up residence in a flat directly opposite and within easy sight of Mr and Mrs Davies's house. Mr Davies senior has had a very long history of mental illness and was retired early as a result. Since coming to Canterbury he has had one fairly long spell in the local mental hospital but seems to have been free of that illness for some time. More recently he has begun to show signs of senile dementia; the neighbours have complained about his noisy movement at night. One day a week he goes to the old people's day centre, and Mrs Davies takes the opportunity to clean and tidy his flat. Mrs Davies's mother is 83 and lives in Scotland. Recently her mother became seriously ill, and in order to be able to go to her Mrs Davies arranged for her father-in-law to spend two weeks resident in the day centre. Unfortunately, he proved very disruptive, and at the time of the interview Mrs Davies was concerned that the day centre would not have him again and that she would not be able to look after her mother should a crisis recur. During the week Mr Davies senior receives his lunch from Meals on Wheels, Age Concern, and the day centre. Unfortunately Mr Davies has recently been asked not to attend Age Concern lunches due to his disruptive behaviour. At the weekends Mrs Davies takes his meals over to him. Mr Davies is bathed at the day centre. Apart from her husband, Mrs Davies lives with two teenage children who are about to leave home to go to university.*

Mrs Evans *is 62 and looks after her 86-year-old mother, who lives with Mr and Mrs Evans. Mrs Evans's mother came to live with her daughter and son-in-law when her husband died twenty-six years ago. At that time Mrs Evans was working part-time but as her mother became increasingly frail so Mrs Evans decided to give up paid work. The old lady has been partially sighted due to cataracts since before her arrival in the Evanses' home but more recently she has become senile. Once a week she goes to the old people's day centre. Two years ago she agreed to spend two weeks there, and her daughter and son-in-law had their first holiday without her for twenty-six years. Since then Mrs Evans's mother has refused to stay overnight in the day centre again, and Mrs Evans has given up trying to persuade her to go. Mr Evans is away a great deal in his job as a sales representative, and their two children have long since left home. Mrs Evans, who is very lonely, would like to travel with her husband on his business trips but is unable to do so because she cannot leave her mother. Apart from the one day at the day centre no other services are received.*

Mrs Fisher *is 69 years old and cares for her husband, who is 59. Twenty-nine years ago, at the age of 31, Mr Fisher had a cerebral haemorrhage and has been brain-damaged ever since. He suffers from very frequent fits, which are at their worst at night, has lost his memory, and is unable to move about except in a wheelchair, which, in the house, he can propel himself. He has recovered some ability to speak, and Mrs Fisher generally understands what he is saying. Just before this catastrophe Mr and Mrs Fisher's son was born, and this son is now adult and has long since left home. Mr and Mrs Fisher have recently moved into a housing trust flat purpose-built for the disabled. Three days a week Mr Fisher spends the day at the local mental hospital and one day a week at the local day centre. Mrs Fisher collects the pensions and does the shopping for a number of her less mobile neighbours. She suffers from arthritis and is concerned about what to do about her 90-year-old mother, who lives in Lancashire and is not at all well. She is worried that she may not see her mother again before she dies. She once tried respite care for her husband at the old people's day centre but felt they had 'muddled his medicine'. Whatever the reason, he had a lot of fits while he was there, and she was reluctant to try respite care again. She is concerned that if she asked for temporary care at the local mental hospital, so that she might visit her mother, the hospital might insist on taking Mr Fisher permanently, which she does not want. Her son has offered to take his father for a week, but she does not consider her son's house suitable.*

Mrs Green *is 56 and cares for her mother-in-law, who is 83. Mrs Green's mother-in-law came to live with Mr and Mrs Green less than a year ago when her husband died. Mrs Green used to work part-time but gave up work some time ago when she 'could see it coming' that her parents-in-law would need her help in the foreseeable future. Mrs Green says there is nothing at all wrong with her mother-in-law, either mentally or physically: 'She knows where she is and she knows where she's well off.' Her mother-in-law refuses to take a bath on her own and won't let Mrs Green help her. The district nurse now comes once a week to bath the old lady, and Mrs Green senior spends one day a week at Age Concern. Mr and Mrs Green have two children who have long since left home; the grandchildren used to come and stay until Mrs Green senior moved into the spare room.*

Mrs Hall *is 51 and cares for her mother, who is 76. Three years ago Mrs Hall, who is one of five sisters, decided that her mother should not* have another winter in her house and arranged for her to come and live with her and her husband. Mrs Hall works thirty hours a week as a cleaner. Her mother is now suffering from senile dementia, is incontinent day and night, wanders a bit, and has had a short spell in hospital for assessment. Mrs Hall has arthritis and recently spent some time in hospital for an operation on her knee. She still walks with some difficulty and depends on a close neighbour to help her with caring for her mother. The neighbour arrives at the Halls' home at 7.30 a.m., stays until 4 p.m., and has on occasion stayed over all night, particularly when Mrs Hall went into hospital for her knee operation. The neighbour goes with Mrs Hall's mother to the day centre which she attends once a week and while there the neighbour helps out with the other old people. The neighbour does all the washing and cleaning up created by the old lady's incontinence. Mrs Hall pays her neighbour, who is a pensioner, the attendance allowance. Apart from the day a week at the day centre, Mrs Hall and her neighbour receive no other assistance. The neighbour was present at the interview and on all subsequent occasions when I visited Mrs Hall.

Mrs Ingram is 65 and cares for her husband, who is also 65. About six years ago, when her husband was still working, he began to show the symptoms of senile dementia. He retired early, and Mr and Mrs Ingram moved from the Midlands to Canterbury – a town they had long before decided they would like to retire to but where they knew virtually no one. Neither of them was told the prognosis for Mr Ingram's illness. Since then he has steadily deteriorated and has now more or less lost the use of all his faculties including speech. Five years ago Mrs Ingram gave up a part-time teaching job to care for her husband. They have one son, who has emigrated. Within the past year Mrs Ingram has herself had a brief spell in hospital. Since then the district nurse has come twice daily to get her husband up and put him to bed in the evening. She also has home help twice a week, and her husband spends one day a week at the day centre.

Mrs Jackson is 56 and is caring for her mother-in-law, who is 91. Mrs Jackson used to teach part-time but gave up three years ago when she needed an operation for which she knew she would have to have a period of convalescence. At the same time, she thought it was time her mother-in-law came to live with her and her husband, since her mother-in-law had just had her first stroke and was having considerable difficulty maintaining herself in her house in London. Since the older Mrs

Jackson has come to live with her son and daughter-in-law, she has had another stroke and has more or less lost her ability to speak. In order to communicate with the family, the old lady writes everything down. There is nothing at all wrong with her mentally, and she can walk short distances with the help of a Zimmer frame. Mr and Mrs Jackson pay for a speech therapist to come once a week, she goes to the day centre once a week, and the district nurse comes once a week to give her a bath. Two of the Jackson children are still in full-time education but come home only for university vacations. Mrs Jackson feels that once all her children have left home the household will be demonstrably 'inefficient', since there will be two adults looking after one very old lady and a dog.

Mrs Knowles is 47 and cares for her mother, who is 79. Her mother has lived with Mr and Mrs Knowles for the past thirteen years and first came to live with them when, due to severe osteoarthritis, she could no longer climb the stairs in her own house. She had been widowed for seven years by then and was lonely. Since the old lady has come to live with them, the Knowles family have moved twice, from one end of the country to the other, and each time the Knowles have bought a house which could provide a 'granny annexe'. The old lady is now, for all practical purposes, blind and, since spending a month in hospital because she fell and broke her hip, she has become somewhat confused. Before her children were born Mrs Knowles was a radiographer and she would now like to re-start her career, since all her children have more or less left home. At present she works part-time and in a voluntary capacity but wants to go on a full-time refresher course for radiography. However, her mother refuses to go to the day centre or to Age Concern for the day and also refuses to stay anywhere else (for example, with another daughter) so that the Knowles family can go on holiday to-gether. District nurses come three times a week to give the old lady a bath, and the GP calls in quite often for an informal chat which Mrs Knowles very much appreciates.

Mrs Lee is 37, and her mother is 70. Mrs Lee's mother has had arthritis for ten years but more recently had a serious heart attack and was in hospital for two weeks. She now has difficulty breathing. Her daughter has borrowed a wheelchair which she uses to take her mother out. During the interview Mrs Lee made it clear on numerous occasions that she did not consider herself to be her mother's primary carer. In her opinion her mother's primary carer is her father; he is over 70 and becoming a little confused himself. However, he does a lot of the housework and the smaller shopping. Mrs Lee works part-time in the mornings only, and every afternoon looks in on her parents, who live five minutes' walk away, to see how they are getting on. She does their bigger shopping and all their washing. Her mother is becoming more and more possessive of Mrs Lee, who is her only child, and Mrs Lee feels increasingly guilty if she and her family go out without her parents. Mrs Lee is worried about the future. If anything happens to either of her parents she doesn't feel that she would welcome either survivor as a permanent resident in her house. Her only contact with the Social Services has been to ask for a reclining chair for her mother (the doctor had suggested this), but Social Services were unable to help. When her mother first came out of hospital her parents had had a home help once a week, but they decided that rather than pay the charge of £1.50 Mrs Lee's father could do the housework.

Mrs Mitchell is 52; her husband is 77. Her husband has arteriosclerosis, and the first sign of his illness was when he turned to his wife three years ago and asked her who she was. Over the past three years Mr Mitchell has passed through most of the stages of senile dementia including considerable wandering, and is now speechless, immobile, and incontinent. Mr Mitchell used to go to the day centre four times a week, but since he developed a urine infection he has stopped going. The district nurse now comes three times a week to bath him, and Social Services have provided special bedding and incontinence pads. At this stage in his illness, Mrs Mitchell feels free to leave her husband alone in the house for brief periods and visit one or other of her adult children, two of whom live near by. Mr Mitchell did spend a week in the local mental hospital but while there he lost a stone in weight, and Mrs Mitchell feels that she herself must care for him until he dies, otherwise she will feel extremely guilty. Mrs Mitchell has primarily been the mother of seven children and, apart from one brief period, has not had a job since she married. While she says she has plans for when her husband dies, she also says that she doesn't know what she will do when she doesn't have to look after him any more.

Miss Nicholson is 61, and her mother, who lives in a 'granny annexe' specially built on to Miss Nicholson's house, is 88. Three years ago Miss Nicholson, her unmarried sister of 59, and her brother decided that the time had come when their mother should no longer live alone. It was also decided that Miss Nicholson had the accommodation most suited to extension and that the annexe for her mother could most easily be built on to her house. When she moved to live with her older daughter the elderly Mrs Nicholson was simply frail; but since arriving in Canterbury she has had five strokes and at one time had thirteen weeks in hospital. While still mentally alert, she now has considerable physical difficulties and is in a wheelchair most of the time. The two Miss Nicholsons share the tasks for caring for their mother almost equally. Every week the other Miss Nicholson travels over 100 miles to stay with her mother and take over all the caring for her for a period of three days. The older Miss Nicholson cares for her mother the other four days of the week. On her days 'off' caring for her mother, Miss Nicholson works as a medical receptionist. Two district nurses come every morning and evening to get the old lady up and to put her to bed again.

Mrs Osborne *is 76, and her husband is 80. Long before they met and married, Mr Osborne had polio and as a result was totally paralysed and confined to a wheelchair. He and his wife met when he was in hospital and she was a nurse. Mrs Osborne has cared for her husband throughout their married life. They have no children. Mrs Osborne used to work part-time in a shop, and Mr Osborne did a great deal of voluntary work although he has not had paid employment since he contracted polio in 1926. In the last ten years Mr Osborne's health has deteriorated. He now has painful arthritis, and his back is giving way. He used to be able to get about in an electric wheelchair, but two years ago he failed the test and has been given nothing to replace it. His wife finds his push-wheelchair too heavy to push very far, and so Mr Osborne is now largely confined to their council flat specially designed for the disabled. Social Services have provided various aids for the physically handicapped in the flat itself, but so far the DHSS has not provided the attendant driven electric wheelchair they long for. Since Mr Osborne developed a urine infection the district nurse comes once a week in order, as Mr Osborne put it, 'to see if I'm still alive!' For a while they had a home help, but decided that there were so many restrictions on what she could do that it wasn't worth having her. Mr Osborne would like his wife to have a rest and is trying to persuade her to allow him to spend a week or two in the old people's day centre. She is reluctant for him to go there, largely on the grounds that most of the other elderly people attending the day centre are mentally confused, whereas Mr Osborne is perfectly all right mentally.*

The men carers

Mr Young *is 84, and his wife is 82. Until his retirement Mr Young was a carpenter. He and his wife have no children. Two years ago they were the first residents to move into a small block of Housing Department wardened flatlets and they are extremely pleased with this accommodation. About eighteen months ago Mrs Young had a series of strokes, and spent some considerable time in hospital. She is now at home, mainly confined to a wheelchair. Her speech and mental agility have both been adversely affected by her strokes. Mr Young is very fit considering his age and can often be seen pushing his wife out in her wheelchair for a walk in central Canterbury. He and his wife have their lunch in the canteen of the flatlets; two district nurses come twice a day every day to get Mrs Young up and put her to bed again; they have home help twice a week; their doctor holds his surgery once a week in the flats; and the warden of the flats is a trained nurse. In an informal conversation with the warden, she told me that she considered the care that the old people get in these flats to be equivalent to 'Part two and a half' (i.e. very like the full-scale public sector residential care provided under Part III of the National Assistance Act, 1947) and that within the past year she herself had had to care for nine residents who had been terminally ill and whom the local geriatric hospital had refused to admit on the grounds that, given that she is a qualified nurse, the flatlets already had the necessary medical staff.*

Mr Williams *is 77 years old. Between making the appointment to interview him and the interview itself Mr Williams's wife, for whom he had been caring, died at the age of 70. Nevertheless, Mr Williams wanted to be interviewed and welcomed the opportunity to talk about his wife's illness and what he had done for her over the past thirteen years. His wife had had a mental disorder which was never apparently diagnosed properly but it meant that, among other things, in fits and starts and over a long period, she lost whole chunks of vocabulary. For four years before her death she had been unable to speak at all. Her physical mobility was also adversely affected but not to the extent that she was unable to go out; indeed Mr Williams had made a point of taking her with him to all sorts of functions including concerts and public lectures. More recently, long absences from home had been curtailed by his wife's incontinence. Mr and Mrs Williams had one son, who was now resident abroad. Despite his wife's death, Mr Williams intended to continue to play an active part in the Carers' Support*

Group, and he is pleased to be called 'a carer' since that is what he used to do in a full-time capacity. He regarded the district nurse who used to visit his wife three times a week as a 'personal friend'. His wife had not worked throughout their marriage.

Mr Vaughan is 76, and his wife, whom he cares for, is 73. Seventeen years ago Mrs Vaughan was diagnosed as having Parkinson's disease, and since then her mobility has considerably deteriorated, so that she now finds it virtually impossible to walk outside the house. Mr Vaughan is himself not well and has recently had a heart attack which adds to his problems of arthritis and long-standing TB. He very often has to go into hospital. Mr and Mrs Vaughan moved to Canterbury quite recently when they found a flat designed for disabled people which they now lease from a housing trust. Before moving, Mr Vaughan had contacted the Social Services to warn them of their imminent arrival. Mr and Mrs Vaughan pay for a companion for Mrs Vaughan who sits with her for four mornings and five evenings a week. They get a home help from Social Services twice a week, and Mrs Vaughan goes to the day centre once a week. Mr Vaughan is very concerned about his wife's future, particularly if he dies before her. He does not want her to go into a home, and she doesn't want to, either, but it looks as though there might be little alternative. Both of them are active mentally and enjoy reading and listening to the radio together. Mrs Vaughan gave up paid work on marriage and had cared for her own mother for five years before she died.

Mr Unwin is 69; his wife, for whom he cares, is 70. For the past five years Mrs Unwin has suffered from senile dementia, and at the time of the interview Mr Unwin had just contacted his doctor to tell him that he couldn't go on caring for his wife at home any longer. He said he was hoping that she would be admitted to the local mental hospital on a permanent basis but that she could come home for temporary stays occasionally. His wife's condition seemed to get worse when they moved from a council house into a one-bedroom flat on the ground floor a few doors away. He felt that his wife had never really adjusted to or understood her new surroundings. Due to the flat's size he and his wife had to sleep in the same room, although he would have preferred not to because of his wife's disturbed sleeping patterns. Apart from the atten- dance allowance, Mr Unwin gets no formal help at all. Two of his daughters live very near him and they occasionally help him bath their mother. During the interview no less than three grandchildren looked in to see their grandparents, but one of these families was about to move some considerable distance away. Mrs Unwin used to go to the day centre once a fortnight but she hated it. Mr Unwin had got to the point where he used to dread the arguments before she went so he stopped sending her there.

DEMOGRAPHIC CHARACTERISTICS OF THE CARERS AND THEIR CARED FOR

Apart from the one constant of residence in Canterbury, every respondent in this small sample had a different story to tell. Among other things, they differed considerably in the length of time that they had been caring and the degree of dependency of the person they were caring for. Some of the people they were caring for were particularly demanding both emotionally and physically, whereas others were keen to give their carers a rest whenever the could.

One of the most interesting variations between them, to my mind, was very large disparities in the services they were receiving from the Social Services Department. It is often claimed that there are gender differences in receipt of social services, such that men carers are more likely to receive formal help than women carers (Bebbington and Davies 1983). Certainly some large data sets seem to indicate this. My own hunch, arising out of this small sample, is that there are at least as important *class* differences, with middle-class men and women carers receiving much more help than working-class men or women carers. The picture is further complicated by the willingness of particular GPs to fight for services for their patients. It was clear from what the respondents told me in this study that some GPs were extremely good at getting services, whereas others – particularly, in this instance, a GP serving a run-down council estate – seemed totally uninterested. Moreover, some services are 'passports' or 'gateways' to other services; living in a Housing Department wardened flatlet is apparently an excellent way of gaining access to a wide range of services, and attending the day centre is a route to a meal and a bath on the day attended. Attendance at Carers' Support Group meetings is at least a way of gaining the ear of a local social worker, occupational therapist, or community

psychiatric nurse, and certainly enables both carers and professionals to put faces to names. Since those attending Support
Group meetings seem, at least at first glance, to be predomi-
nantly middle class, this may be another means whereby class
differences in receipt of services are reinforced. Whether, in
a larger and randomly drawn sample, such class differences
would once again emerge, and whether such tentative indica-
tions of some of their determinants would be established as
valid, can be established only through another, much more
broadly based, and much more expensive research project.

Even with this small sample there are nevertheless certain
demographic characteristics of the carers and cared for that can
be crudely quantified and summarized thereby. Such demographic characteristics of the carers in this small sample can tell
us nothing about the *incidence* of these characteristics in the
general population of carers, either nationally or within the
Canterbury area. However, as I shall argue in the following
chapters, the age, sex, and marital status of both carers and their
cared for are the end-product of important social processes in-
volving material factors, ideology about sex and gender and
about the nature of kinship obligations, negotiation within kinship networks, and, finally, complicated feelings between carers
and their cared for based on personal biography and family
history. But before turning to a discussion of these more general
issues, it is necessary to provide the demographic data on which
some of this discussion in subsequent chapters will be based.

Age, sex, and marital status of the sample

Of the nineteen carers interviewed, fifteen were women and
four were men. All the men were caring for their wives, whereas
eleven of the women were caring for someone other than their
husband – usually a relative from the older generation (see *Table
2*). All the men carers were aged over 65, and one of the men, at
84, was the oldest carer in the group. In contrast, as one would
expect given that it was only women who were caring for someone of a different generation from themselves, the women's
ages spread over a much wider age range, with the youngest
under 40 and the oldest in her late seventies. *Table 1* summarizes
the ages and sex of the carers and cared for, and *Table 2* their kin
relationship.

Table 1 Ages and sex of carers and cared for

	carers			cared for	
	men	women		men	women
under 50	—	4		—	—
50–60	—	6		1	—
60–65	—	2		—	—
65–70	1	2		1	—
70–75	—	—		—	3
75–80	2	1		2	5
80–85	1	—		1	3
85 plus	—	—		1	3
Total	4	15		6	14[1]

[1] Includes one woman being cared for by a carer of two people.

Table 2 Kin relationship between carers and cared for

child of cared for		child-in-law of cared for		spouse of cared for		other	
men	women	men	women	men	women	men	women
—	7	—	4	4	4	—	1[1]

[1] Includes one woman being cared for by a carer of two people.

These tables immediately show that there were considerable differences between the men and women carers in terms of their ages and the variety (or lack of it) of their kin relationships with the people they were caring for. Indeed, there are such interesting differences – for example, that all the men carers were looking after their wives, whereas most of the women were caring for someone in the older generation – that it is tempting to draw some conclusions about the different kinds of caring that men and women *in general* do. With such a small and unrepresentative sample, this would be an illegitimate thing to do. However, in the following three chapters – Chapter 3 on becoming a carer, Chapter 4 on a life-cycle typology of carers, and Chapter 5 on the reasons for caring – I will occasionally suggest that these differences may well recur in a general population because there seem to be wider social processes which have, to a significant extent, determined how these nineteen people emerged as carers.

Before turning to the study of these particular nineteen carers in detail, it is necessary to establish that I did interview the right person, i.e. that the demographic characteristics described above exhaustively cover all the carers of the people being cared for. In other words, were there any people in this group of cared for who were being cared for by more than one person to such an extent that it is possible to describe the caring as 'joint' with another person or persons? Did I in fact omit to interview some crucial carers? It is to this question that I now turn.

'JOINT' CARING?

Who exactly constitutes a 'carer' is a question of definition. Some of the problems of definition, particularly with reference to this sample, have already been referred to. Partly the definitional problems arise out of the concept of 'caring', as instanced in the example of the carer who greeted me with the words, 'I'm a *daughter*, not a carer!'. However, there are also problems of definition surrounding what a carer actually *does*. Is a 'carer' only someone who does intimate caring tasks for a highly dependent person, or does one include as a 'carer' someone who does a lot of housework for an elderly person but no more intimate tasks? In this small sample, and with access to a very particular universe, I simply took what I was given and used the interview irrespective of what the respondent actually did and without any preordained definition of what constituted a 'proper' carer. (This is, in my opinion, somewhat sloppy and certainly not a procedure to be followed with a larger sample where one would need some control over quantitative data. With such a small sample as here, I do not think it matters too much, and the variation in what the 'carers' did was in itself interesting and is discussed further in Chapter 6.) As it happens, with this sample there were only three 'carers' whose only work – as yet – was housework, and all the others were faced with tasks of varying degrees of intimacy. However, one or two of the respondents were themselves aware that there was a problem about definition. In the clearest case, Mrs Lee denied that she was the 'carer' and claimed that her father was 'really' the carer of her mother. In another case, Mrs Archer, it became clear during the interview that Mrs Archer's husband was of the opinion that his father-in-law was the 'carer' of Mrs Archer's rather sick mother but he thought that his father-in-law was making an unnecessarily bad job of it and hence that his wife was being coerced through anxiety and guilt into doing far more for her mother than was 'really' needed. (Both these cases are discussed in much more detail in Chapter 3; they seemed to be caring relationships that were in an early stage of development and still subject to negotiation within a kin network.) In neither case did I interview the other 'carer' who members of these two families claimed was pre-eminent. Secondly, there were three carers who were quite happy with that description of themselves but who, when I came to look at what someone else in their circle did for their dependent relative, could be considered to be in a 'joint' caring situation.

Before turning to a discussion of these three joint carers, it is interesting to look at the other respondents to see if, particularly where a married woman was caring for her own parent or, more especially, one of her husband's parents, husband and wife could be described as 'joint' carers. The answer is emphatically negative. None of the wives suggested that their husbands made any major contribution to the caring they did. In two cases (Mrs Jackson and Mrs Green, both of whom were caring for their mothers-in-law) the husbands were present in the house during the interviews, but at no point were they asked by their wives to participate in the interviews. Many of the wives said their husbands were 'very good'. By this they seemed to mean that their husbands rarely complained and sometimes gave them strong moral support. Some of the wives felt distinctly guilty about what their husbands had to put up with (a point developed further in Chapter 6). None of the husbands seemed to do very much of a practical nature (apart from Mr Cook, who bathed his father-in-law when he stayed with them), and in one or two cases the husbands took considerable avoiding action. (see Chapter 6 for a fuller discussion of why the husbands seemed to have particular difficulty about caring for their own parents.)

This lack of contribution by husbands of married women

carers has been very well documented in other studies, particularly that by Nissel and Bonnerjea (1982). However, before leaping to some jaundiced opinions concerning the contribution, or lack of it, that husbands make to the care of their own or their wives' parents, it is important to remember two things. First, in this study none of the wives thought their husbands could have done more than they did; and without exception the wives took it for granted that it was their husbands' task to provide financially for their families, including, where necessary, the financial resources needed for the care of the elderly dependent person. Given that many of the wives were providing almost constant care, the contribution the husbands would have had to make, if the caring were to come near to 'joint' care, was very considerable. Secondly, all the husbands, bar one, were in full-time paid work, and some of them were very well paid. If they had given up full-time paid work to take on the occupation of unpaid caring, the standard of living of all these families would have been very much reduced, and the social status of both wives and husbands would have taken a very hard knock. (Such material factors in the determination of who cares are discussed further in Chapter 4.)

To return to the three carers whom I assess as being in an established 'joint' arrangement: these were Mrs Hall, Mr Vaughan, and Miss Nicholson. Interestingly, in all three cases, the other carer was a woman. Mrs Hall and Mr Vaughan were each paying someone to give them very substantial amounts of help; indeed, in the case of Mrs Hall, the paid carer was probably doing as much (if not more) for Mrs Hall's mother as Mrs Hall herself – at least, during the day. The fact that Mrs Hall and Mr Vaughan were apparently employing a joint carer might imply some similarity between them; in fact their two caring arrangements could hardly have been more different. Mrs Hall was using her mother's attendance allowance to pay an old-age pensioner who lived opposite her on the same council estate to do a great deal of the caring for her mother. Basically the 'joint' carer was in the Halls' house from 7.30 a.m. to 4 p.m. every day, and Mrs Hall went out to work part-time. Mrs Hall and her neighbour were old friends, and although the arrangement had a contractual element to it, it was based on affection and solidarity between these two women. In contrast, Mr Vaughan's private arrangement had been made with a stranger recommended to him by the SSD. A qualified nurse came and sat with his wife for five evenings and four mornings a week, largely to provide his wife with what he described as the kind of 'feminine' companionship he felt he could not himself provide for her. This paid companion also did some of the housework, including ironing and washing-up, but apparently little actual nursing. The chief purpose seemed to be to allow Mr Vaughan some time to himself, which was otherwise subject to constant interruption from his wife, to allow him to pursue his own interests in reading and painting. In neither case did I seek to interview the other carer. Both these other carers were in some sense 'employed' and hence fell rather more into the conventional view of what constitutes 'formal' rather than 'informal' caring. Given that this study was about 'informal' caring, this fact seemed at the time reason enough for ignoring the other carer. I saw Mrs Hall on a number of occasions, and each time the other carer was with her; indeed, the other carer was there throughout my formal interview with Mrs Hall, and the interview itself had considerable joint elements to it. Hence I felt that, in a sense, I had gathered at least a minimum understanding of the motivation of Mrs Hall's friend and neighbour.

Both Mrs Hall and Mr Vaughan were using their additional paid help for somewhat similar purposes. Both of them wanted time to develop their own interests and maintain as much a semblance of normality as possible. But there the similarities between them ended; in terms of context, the social and economic differences between them were very considerable, and the way they had gone about finding a joint carer also had a strong class difference about it. In Mr Vaughan's case, his relationship with the joint carer was a hierarchical one and closely followed the model of employer/employee. In Mrs Hall's case, her relationship with the paid joint carer was not at all hierarchical and most closely followed the model of friendship. However, there is no doubt the attendance allowance was very important in generating this help for Mrs Hall. Both these cases also indicated that, where there are additional resources to pay for it, the payment of an additional carer may be the sufficient (and necessary?) condition for the maintenance of an otherwise informal caring relationship.

The third case of 'joint' caring concerned an elaborate arrangement made between two unmarried sisters. Miss Nicholson was
quite clear that she was a 'joint' carer with her sister who travelled
a long distance each week in order to live in Miss Nicholson's
house and devote herself to caring for their mother for three full
days. At the time they had made this arrangement neither of the
sisters had been in paid work of any kind, but since they had
reached this agreement the older Miss Nicholson, in whose
house their mother lived, had taken the opportunity to work
two full days as a medical receptionist. This arrangement
had been made formally between the sisters and their younger
brother. Their brother was the person who had really organized
it; it was he who had been delegated to ask their mother what
she herself thought was best. However, it had never been on the
agenda that their mother might go to her son. Miss Nicholson
explained this in terms of the additional calls on his time of his
paid job, his children, and his wife. The brother was now a
regular visitor to Miss Nicholson's home to see his mother, and
he had arranged for their mother to stay in a residential home
near him in London in order to give the two Miss Nicholsons a
holiday, but that had been the extent of his practical help. He
seems to have been more of a broker of the family's caring
resources rather than a caring resource himself. In this case, I
made no effort to contact the other Miss Nicholson, and so a
potential contact with a 'joint' informal carer was lost.

Thus, to conclude this chapter, it is clear that there are certain
dificulties about this sample. It was highly self-selected, not
based on any clear definition of what constitutes a 'carer', and in
five known cases (I here include the fathers of Mrs Lee and Mrs
Archer) did not properly cover the other 'joint' carer. Nevertheless, it seems to me that this very 'raggedyness' has the potential
to throw up some interesting contrasts and colours. We now
turn to an analysis and discussion of the interviews.

3
Becoming a carer:
the negotiation process

In the next three chapters I attempt to elucidate the social processes that created the caring relationships of the nineteen
carers in the study. The simple question that I have in mind is,
Why did this particular individual become a carer? In other
words, and immediately to make the question more complicated, what were the social, psychological, ideological, material,
and historical processes which brought these particular caring
relationships into existence? Also, were these processes gendered in some way and, if so, how?

To answer such nigh impossible questions pitched at such a pro-
found level of generality, it is necessary to reduce them once more
to some simpler formulation and one that is easier to handle
with the data from this study. In this chapter, in order to begin
to develop an understanding of why each of these carers became
a carer, I shall examine whether or not there were *alternative*
sources of care available to the person they were caring for – that
is, how far it was the case, as some of the carers themselves
claimed, that they were the 'obvious person' to take on the care
of the particular dependent elderly person in question.

In order to assess these possible alternatives, it is necessary to
make assumptions about the kind of alternative to which the
carers might themselves look. There are various ways of formu-
lating such alternatives. Particularly with reference to the kin

network, Hazel Qureshi (Qureshi and Walker, forthcoming) has recently developed a ranking of kin with a very high level of predictability. In her ranking, very close female kin are much the most likely to be called on first. In this study, the carers themselves often referred to possible alternative carers within their immediate kin network, usually to explain why these particular relatives could not have taken on the full caring responsibility. Frequently they also mulled over the possibility of a more formal kind of care. These alternatives can be summarized as follows:

(1) *Informal care* provided by someone else in the very close kin network of the person being cared for. In the case of a spouse caring for their husband or wife, such alternative carers might be drawn from the married couple's own children. In the case of carers caring for someone in the older generation, particularly their own parent or parent-in-law, the alternative carers might be drawn from the carer's own siblings or siblings-in-law.

(2) *Formal care* on a permanent and full-time basis, from either the public or the private sector. Such care was often referred to by the carers in this study as 'putting someone in a home' or 'putting her away'. One variation on this full-time substitute for informal care is a wardened flatlet – a form of residential care on a less than full-time basis to which only one of the carers in this sample referred.

In this chapter I shall concentrate on the kin networks of carer and cared for. (The question of permanent full-time residential care is largely considered in Chapter 5 within the context of a more general discussion of love and guilt.) *Table 3* summarizes the hypothetical *informal* alternatives of the nineteen carers in the sample. Much of this information on the close kin of the person being cared for was systematically collected, although by the time I reached these questions the carers themselves had usually already told me a great deal about their kin particularly when explaining how it was that they had emerged as 'the' carer. What is particularly interesting about this data is that in every case the *marital status* of immediate *male* kin was always volunteered by the carer respondent. I never asked for this information. In other words, *all* the respondents were at some pains to point out whether or not a male blood relative had a *wife* who might be an alternative carer. While occasionally I was told, in passing, the marital status of female kin, this was by no means universal, so I am not able to include these data here. The point about the importance of female kin by marriage is one that we shall return to in the discussion of the carers' own views about possible alternative carers.

Table 3 demonstrates two kinds of proximity and distance: proximity of kinship – especially female kinship – and geographical proximity or geographical distance. In both kinds of relation, it is often rather difficult to see why these particular carers had emerged from these particular networks, except perhaps in the case of the carers looking after their own spouses (and even here there are one or two puzzles which are discussed later in this chapter).

The three carers who were only children, or whose husbands were only children, had no immediate kin network to call on. For them there had been little alternative for their elderly relative except some more formal kind of residential care. But for some of the other carers, particularly those with large numbers of siblings, there seems to have been some determining factor other than particular proximity of kinship or even geographical proximity. For example, if we look at those with sisters, there were five women caring for their mothers (or, in the case of Mrs Archer, for both parents) who had sisters; admittedly, of these five cases, Miss Nicholson's sister had shouldered more or less half of the caring task (see Chapter 2), while Mrs Evans's sister was really out of the running since she had married a man from Eastern Europe and now lived there. But Mrs Hall was one of five sisters, three of whom lived in or near Canterbury. One of these was already a carer of her disabled husband, but the remaining two were in the same position as Mrs Hall – married and with grown-up families. Mrs Knowles, who was not Canterbury born, had twice moved with her mother up and down the length of the country, but neither of her sisters had ever been their mother's carer. One of these sisters had been very seriously ill for many years and, at the time of the interview, had recently died. Mrs Archer's sister lived within half an hour's easy drive of Canterbury.

In the case of Mrs Hall and Mrs Knowles, a major determining factor seems to have been their idea that, of all the sisters

Table 3 Alternative carers in the immediate kin network

caring for own mother	
Mrs K.	2 sisters (1 recently dead after long disabling illness; 1 living in north of England)
Mrs H.*	4 sisters (1 in Australia; 1 with a disabled husband; 2 living locally)
Mrs E.	1 sister (in Eastern Europe); 1 brother (married and living in Midlands)
Miss N.	1 sister (joint carer); 1 brother (married and living in London)
caring for own father (and aunt)	
Mrs C.*	1 brother (married and living locally); aunt has no living children, husband still alive
caring for a parent-in-law	
Mrs D.	husband an only child
Mrs G.	husband an only child
Mrs B.*	husband has 1 brother, now separated from wife
Mrs J.	husband has 3 brothers (1 in Australia; 1 widowed and living in West Country; 1 married and living in family home in Ireland)
caring for both parents	
Mrs A.*	1 sister (resident elsewhere in Kent); 1 brother (married, living in East Anglia)
Mrs L.*	an only child
caring for a husband	
Mrs F.	1 son, married, living elsewhere in Kent
Mrs I.	1 son, married, living in New Zealand
Mrs M.	4 sons (2 married); 3 daughters
Mrs O.	no children
caring for a wife	
Mr U.	2 sons; 1 daughter from Mrs U.'s previous marriage (all now out of touch with their mother); 3 daughters; 1 son from Mr and Mrs U's marriage (2 daughters live very close; 1 daughter in Australia; son separated from wife and out of touch)
Mr V.	2 daughters (both living in other parts of the country)
Mr W.	1 son (unmarried, living in North America)
Mr Y.	no children

*These five carers care for a parent or parents who have always lived in Canterbury, and the carers themselves have never left Canterbury (apart from Mrs L., who was, until her husband's recent retirement from the local Canterbury regiment, an army wife travelling with him world-wide). In other words, in these five cases neither carer nor cared for has had to move towards each other. All the other carers of parents or parents-in-law have had to make special arrangements to gain proximity.

involved in these kin networks, Mrs Hall and Mrs Knowles were the ones most suited to the care of this particular elderly person. For example, Mrs Hall was proud of the fact that she had been the one historically closest to her mother:

'We've been so close. I was the favourite. Mum and Dad would never turn up unasked on the other sisters' doorstep. But she would come here.'

One of Mrs Hall's two sisters who could equally have been their mother's carer had always been of the firm opinion that their mother should be in a 'home', while the other had initially offered to have their mother, 'but then Mother said she wanted to come to me'. Thus, in this case Mrs Hall seems to have emerged as the carer in this network because of mutual affection between the daughter and her mother. However, although the idea that both her mother and herself had preferred this arrangement was a source of comfort, she nevertheless felt that her sisters had unfairly landed her with all the responsibility:

'My sisters could definitely help more – they could give me a rest. They say she should be in a home. They don't want to be bothered.'

Mrs Knowles also seems to have emerged as her mother's carer because of some special features of their relationship, although in this case it was less that they were particularly fond of each other (see page 120) but rather that her mother and her one able-bodied sister did not get on very well; Mrs Knowles seemed to be the lesser of two evils:

'Mother doesn't like her very much – it's a long-standing dislike. She's a nurse and she's terribly *bustly*. That's another reason why she didn't care for Granny.'

An additional reason in this particular case was that, at the time when it was becoming obvious that their mother was going blind, this sister 'wasn't married and didn't have the facilities to look after her. She was living in rented accommodation.' In other words, Mrs Knowles perceived there to be material conditions to the selection of a suitable carer within the kin network, and this sister did not fulfil those conditions. Her second sister was already ill with the disabling illness that led to her premature death.

Mrs Archer's selection as carer within the kin network, despite having a sister living in a nearby town (and a married brother living in East Anglia), seemed on the surface to be the most straightforward self-selection due to geographical proximity. But on closer inspection this was probably one of the most interesting examples of a caring relationship in an early and fluctuating state (the Archers are discussed in more detail later on). Unlike with Mrs Hall and Mrs Knowles, Mrs Archer's parents still lived in their own household. The ostensible reason for Mrs Archer's selection as 'the' carer was that her parents lived in Canterbury and so did she. During the interview Mrs Archer more than once pointed out that she and her husband had always lived within a few hundred yards of her parents – at which point Mr Archer, who was present throughout the interview, interjected that they lived 'too close'. When I asked her if there were any problems about caring for her parents, Mr Archer replied:

'It's inconveniences more than difficulties. We get the brunt of it because we happen to live in Canterbury unfortunately.'

Mrs Archer told me of the difficulty she had in passing by the end of the street where her parents lived on her way to and from work every day, and how she had to resist going in to see them more than her regular three times a week. She said that her bother, who lived in East Anglia, gave her unheedable advice:

'My brother says, "Oh, only go down once a week." But I can't do that.'

Thus in this case geographical proximity seemed to be not so much the determining factor in deciding who should care in a particular network, but rather the fertilizer for guilt in the mind of the geographically nearest daughter and the generator of the idea that someone needed caring for at all. When I asked Mrs Archer whether she thought others could help more than they did, she said:

'Sometimes I get bitter to my sister – but we're not the best of friends!'

And Mr Archer interjected bitterly, 'You can't change people, can you! My sister-in-law views it clinically. My brother-in-law's wife views it clinically too.'

This comment from Mr Archer seems to me particularly interesting on two counts. First, he seemed to be saying that, in the case of his wife, geographical proximity and feeling for her parents fed upon each other; secondly, he was also saying – like all the other respondents – that, in a kin network, brothers did not count as alternatives, *but their wives did*. It is this point concerning brothers and the access that they gave to a second-ary ranking of female kin – the sisters-in-law – that we turn to now.

Brothers and brothers-in-law did not seem to feature for any of the carers as possible alternative carers. These men could, if they were married, however, provide access to a sister-in-law as an alternative carer. Mrs Evans and Miss Nicholson both had brothers; but they both had entirely discounted these men as possible alternative carers, particularly on the grounds of their brothers' careers. Yet there was some degree of feeling on the part of both these women (especially Mrs Evans, who was really quite bitter) that their sisters-in-law might have done more than they did, particularly to give them some short respite:

'I know my brother feels guilty that he does so little – but he has got a *wife*. . . . His wife has never had her, not even for a holiday. His wife doesn't feel she has to do anything for Mother. . . . I thought my brother might take over after he got his degree but he married soon after and his wife didn't want her.'

Mrs Cook also had a brother whom she discounted as a possible alternative carer on the grounds of his job (he was self-employed) although she thought he could do more gardening for their father at the weekends:

'I sometimes feel that my brother could do more, especially this year with the garden. But then I think that perhaps I'm being selfish. He says, "All right – be a martyr!" We just laugh it off.'

But in contrast to Mrs Evans, Mrs Cook also thought that her sister-in-law (her brother's wife) had been more than helpful when her mother was dying and that she had actually done some of the personal caring tasks that Mrs Cook had herself found difficult to do; her sister-in-law now did the caring work for Mrs Cook's father one day a week. Mrs Archer was the only carer of her own parents who had a brother but also made no reference to the possibility that her sister-in-law might help more (although Mr Archer thought she could; see above). With her there was slightly more of an expectation that her brother might contribute at least some practical help. For ex-ample, talking about her parents' move into an almshouse, she said, 'I *made* my sister and my brother help me with their move.'

Interestingly, and perhaps significantly, of those women caring for their in-laws, not one was caring for someone who had a daughter. It is possible, indeed probable, that if these elderly people had had daughters they would not have called on the services of their daughters-in-law (cf. Qureshi and Walker, forthcoming). But even with this kin by marriage there had ostensibly been alternatives in two cases. Mrs Barnes's mother-in-law had had another daughter-in-law living locally; similarly, Mrs Jackson's mother-in-law, who had moved from London in order to take up residence in the Jacksons' household, apparently could have gone to live with another daughter-in-law who was actually living in the old lady's original home in Ireland. Both Mrs Jackson and Mrs Barnes, like the carers with brothers, discounted their brothers-in-law as alternative carers but regarded their brothers-in-law's wives as legitimate alternative carers. For example, Mrs Jackson, in listing all her husband's brothers (there were three, one of whom was resident in Australia and hence really out of the running) said of the one living in the West Country:

'My mother-in-law tried living with him a few nights. It wasn't a great success. He was widowed about seven years ago and now there's no woman in the house. He thinks Part Three would be the best solution.'

Having eliminated that possibility, the one remaining was the brother living in his mother's original home in Ireland:

'The house is too remote from anywhere, and anyway, she doesn't like that daughter-in-law.'

However, it then emerged that, within the older Mrs Jackson's kin network, there were also four nieces living in the West Country who cared about their aunt. One of them often took care of her when the Jacksons went on holiday:

'She has four nieces in the West Country and she often stays with one of them in particular.'

'Why aren't they her carers?'

'But why should they? She knows them very well – better than she knows me. But I'm the closer relation.'

Thus Mrs Jackson seemed to have an idea, that, within a given ranking of kinship obligations (and she clearly thought that daughters-in-law took precedence over nieces), these ranked obligations were more powerful in the selection of a carer than feelings of affection or other less identifiable forms of proximity.

Mrs Barnes had a similar view that men gave access through marriage to women carers. Early on in the interview she had explained to me:

'My husband has a brother. My sister-in-law has in the past been a great help but she's now separated from my brother-in-law.'

It was in some sense obvious to Mrs Barnes that her sister-in-law had been obligated to help their mother-in-law in the same way as Mrs Barnes herself had by marriage, but that the end of marriage brought that obligation to an end. Admittedly she thought her husband's brother could have done something more than the token visiting he had until recently been willing to do (although even that had fallen by the wayside recently):

'My brother-in-law used to come here twice a week – but he didn't even turn off the car engine! It was just a conscience visit. He's never offered to look after my mother-in-law, and my husband hasn't asked him. It's a situation that you tend to slip into, isn't it really?'

It did indeed seem that Mrs Barnes had 'slipped into' being a carer. Like Mrs Archer, discussed above, geographical proximity had in a sense created Mrs Barnes as 'the' carer rather than her sister-in-law. The wife of the older son, Mrs Barnes lived on the same small estate as her mother-in-law (their houses were within fifty yards of each other). With the onset of senile dementia it became impossible to ignore her mother-in-law's increasingly erratic behaviour, particularly at night. The result was that, to prevent her disturbing the entire family, Mrs Barnes had taken to locking her mother-in-law in her house every night. But this had itself become a problem, since Mrs Barnes had become haunted by the idea that her mother-in-law would set herself or her house on fire and be unable to escape through a locked door:

'We lock her in. No open fires, no matches, no candles. She couldn't get out if there were a fire. It's awful.'

Finally Mrs Barnes had become so anxious about the fact that her mother-in-law lived so close and yet, at night, so inaccessibly that the Barnes family were selling their estate and amalgamating the two households into one house with a 'granny annexe'. Thus in this case very close geographical proximity (arising originally out of a sort of primogeniture) had 'selected' one daughter-in-law rather than another.

The idea that male blood relatives gave access to caring women through their marriages cropped up again and again and was not confined to those women carers who either were 'in-law' carers themselves or had sisters-in-law whom they felt they could legitimately call on for help. Mrs Cook, for example, said with reference to her own eventual care in her own old age:

'There's never quite the same between the boy and the parents and the daughter and the parents. If the son's married I think it falls on the poor wife. She's the one that actually does it.'

And Mrs Archer said, again with reference to caring for herself in her own old age, 'Having two sons, I would need daughters-in-law.'

Thus these carers seemed to share a common view of the nature of kinship obligations and the way that particular kin relations work. All kinship obligations are gendered. Working from that most basic assumption, they all took the view that daughters take precedence over sons; that married sons give access to daughters-in-law; that, where a daughter is the main carer, daughters-in-law can be legitimately called upon to give assistance; and that, where there are no daughters, daughters-in-law are also daughters in lieu. More distant blood relations, such as nieces, do not seem to have nearly as much obligation as daughters-in-law, even if these nieces are on very good and close terms with their elderly aunt. In the one example of a niece carer in this sample, it is perhaps significant that her aunt was her deceased mother's sister. The carer herself – Mrs Cook – explained this in terms of a surrogate mother/daughter relationship:

'I was always very close to my mother. I think in some respects Auntie's taken over Mum's place for me – and my aunt didn't have a daughter. I've become even closer to her now.'

Sometimes these kinship obligations had, in this sample, been reinforced by death-bed pronouncements. For example, to explain her motivation to care for her father, Mrs Cook said:

'Mum said just before she died . . . she said to me, "You will take care of Father, won't you?" And being an only daughter one just automatically does.'

Mrs Green reported that something very similar had happened when her father-in-law was dying:

'My father-in-law said to her when he was dying, "Susan will look after you."'

However, within this common view of the gendered and ranked nature of kinship obligations (which has been confirmed by much larger studies, e.g. Qureshi and Walker, forthcoming), there were certain choices being made that were peculiar to each family. These choices seemed to be based on three features, at least within this small sample. These features were, first, a perception of the quality of the relationship between the carer and the cared for and, where there was a potential choice of women carers of equal kinship ranking, a perception of the relative quality of that relationship; secondly, geographical proximity, but this relatively simple and easily measured concept was probably more complicated since actual proximity seemed in itself to provide the context for the development of strong guilt feelings; and, thirdly, material conditions, particularly where households were being amalgamated: whether, for example, there was 'room' for the elderly person, and whether there were adequate and secure household resources (usually assumed to invoke the assistance of a male bread-winner) to cover the additional expenses of informal care.

So far there has been no discussion of the way a carer spouse emerges as 'the' carer. This is because, at an ideological level in our society, marriage is regarded as the supreme caring relationship, rivalled perhaps only by the mother/infant bond. Marriage vows (to which almost all of the caring spouses referred) act to reinforce the idea that one of the fundamental responsibilities of marriage is to care 'in sickness and in health'. Thus, in a sense, there seems nothing to say about why and how the married carers emerged; they were simply fulfilling their ascribed role as spouses, and to do otherwise would be to threaten the very nature and continuity of their marriages. However, I have suggested above that where a carer is looking after their own spouse, the alternative informal carers within their immediate kin network might be their own children or children-in-law. This might particularly be the case where the caring spouse is himself or herself increasingly elderly and frail. In this sample the spouse carers, particularly the men, were among the oldest carers in the sample (see *Tables 1* and *2*, p. 35). Three of the men carers were over 75, and three of the women carers of their husbands were over 65. Most of these older carers claimed that they were in as good health as could be expected, but two of them (Mr Vaughan and Mrs Ingram) had recently had lengthy spells in hospital for their own chronic ailments. Of the eight spouse carers, for a number of them there was no very obvious alternative carer in their immediate kin network (see *Table 3*, p. 44); two (Mrs Osborne and Mr Young) had had no children, and two had had only sons who had emigrated (Mrs Ingram and Mr Williams). Of the remaining four, Mrs Fisher had an only son who was married and living elsewhere in Kent, but he had been brought up with his father's mental and physical disabilities and still found them, according to Mrs Fisher, rather disturbing. Thus for only three spouse carers was there an obvious source of alternative carers. Mrs Mitchell had seven children, which in terms of female kin amounted to three daughters and two actual or quasi-daughters-in-law; Mr Unwin had four children from his marriage to Mrs Unwin, including two daughters living practically opposite him; Mr Vaughan, who had during his lifetime moved around the Home Counties a good deal, had two daughters living in other parts of southern and eastern England.

Thus five of the spouse carers were relatively isolated in their own immediate kin networks. This in itself might explain why some of them had carried on caring for such considerable lengths of time while they themselves were moving into increasingly frail old age. Of the three spouse carers remaining, one (Mrs Mitchell) was, at fifty-two, the youngest and fittest, and hence perhaps not much in need of the assistance, let alone substitution, of an alternative carer drawn from her large family. The remaining two spouse carers were, however, rather more obvious candidates for alternatives; Mr Unwin had two daughters living practically opposite him, and Mr Vaughan had two daughters with whom he might have been living.

The position of Mr Unwin and Mr Vaughan brings us to the nub of the point of this section of this chapter. In their different ways, both Mr Unwin and Mr Vaughan appeared to be spouse carers who had emerged as the result of a negotiation process, although not necessarily an explicit one. On the very day of the interview one of Mr Unwin's daughters who lived opposite to him was moving to a small seaside town some ten miles from Canterbury. Mr Unwin was extremely upset on two counts; he was losing some of his network of support, which had been based perhaps rather less on his daughter than on her children, and secondly, she had decided to move without consulting him. Mr Unwin clearly felt that she should have considered his needs before such a decision to move away had been taken. In other words, he had assumed that his daughter understood that she was an alternative carer, whereas she was acting as though it was already established that he was the main – and only – carer of her mother. An implicit understanding between father and this daughter, tacit only because very close geographical proximity had meant that there was no need to spell the understanding out, had not in fact existed. Mr Unwin was very abruptly being 'negotiated' into the position of chief carer. His response was to contact his doctor immediately, with a view to having his wife admitted to permanent residential care. Mr Vaughan had also been 'negotiated' into caring for his wife by his two daughters, but in a rather more explicit way; the story of the Vaughans is discussed in much more detail below.

Both the case of Mr Unwin and that of Mr Vaughan seem to me to demonstrate a general truth: namely, that marriage is generally regarded as the pre-eminent caring relationship, except where a husband cares for a wife and there are daughters or daughters-in-law apparently available for caring. In other words, *the obligations of marriage are cross-cut, and can be contradicted, by the obligations of gendered kinship*. Where there is an elderly, dependent, and still married woman, there will, I suggest, always be tension between her husband and any of her daughters or daughters-in-law as to who should shoulder the main responsibility for her care. I have designated this tension, perhaps euphemistically, as 'negotiation'. In this sample, Mr Vaughan had emerged as the settled carer as the result of long and protracted 'negotiation' (see below); Mr Unwin had suddenly discovered that negotiations were involved; and three women carers (Mrs Archer, Mrs Lee, and Mrs Cook) were at various stages in the negotiation process concerning responsibility for the care of a still married dependent woman in their immediate kin network. Let us now consider these three women and Mr Vaughan more closely.

NEGOTIATING A CARER: GENDER AND MARRIAGE

As just mentioned, it seems to me that there is considerable tension between fathers and their close female kin in the younger generation when it comes to deciding who should care for their elderly wives. In this sample, there were three cases where it seemed that an elderly man living with his chronically sick wife was increasingly calling on the aid of an alternative carer. In all three cases the alternative carers were relatively young women, two of them daughters and one of them a niece. Two of these women – both the daughters – were showing considerable signs of tension over this apparent change in their status, while, as I shall suggest below, the niece had reason to be adjusted to this role already.

The two daughters, Mrs Archer and Mrs Lee, were in many ways rather similar. Both had parents who lived close by, and both their mothers were rather ill. At the same time both their fathers were showing increasing signs that they either would not or could not cope with their mothers' illness. Mrs Archer's father had never, according to both Mr and Mrs Archer, lifted a finger in the house. Indeed Mrs Archer said her mother acknowledged that she had spoilt her father – 'to keep the peace, as it were, she's always had dinner on his plate for him'. The domestic scene was summarized by Mr Archer when he described what happened when Mrs Archer's mother had a stroke: 'He sat and finished his tea while she laid in the hearth.' At the same time Mr and Mrs Archer described the father as a man who was increasingly confused and whose moods and long silences were getting worse. Similarly, Mrs Lee's father was also showing signs of mild confusion, but he was quite happy doing the housework; he and his wife had stopped having a home help on the grounds that he could manage. His problem, however, was that he could not face the fact that his wife was ill, and he had refused to travel with her in the ambulance after her heart attack, not once visiting her in hospital. According to Mrs Lee, he was terrified of finding his wife dead.

When interviewing Mrs Lee and especially Mrs Archer it was

often difficult to know whether they were more worried and 'caring' about their mother or their father. (On the form all the respondents returned saying they were willing to be interviewed, Mrs Archer had named both her parents as the people she was caring for.) Clearly in both these situations of a caring relationship between elderly spouses where the carers were elderly men, the caring relationships were beginning to break down. In their place, new caring relationships between parents and the daughters were assuming greater importance.

However, these new relationships were subject to negotiation, not only between the parents and the daughters, but also between the other interested parties competing for the daughters' services: namely, the daughters' husbands and their children. In the case of Mr and Mrs Archer, who were interviewed together, Mr Archer was very articulate about his needs in relation to those of his parents-in-law. He was keen that his wife do less for her parents than she was already doing, arguing that 'we've tried to make them as self-reliant as possible; we are the long-stop' and suggesting to his wife that it was necessary for her to see her parents only once a week rather than the three times a week she currently saw them. He said, with some resentment, that his parents-in-law were reluctant to accept the help of the Social Services Department, and he mimicked them, saying, 'Don't bother to do that – *Gillian* will do it.' At that he turned to his wife and said, 'You've enough to do in our own house without cleaning other people's!'

Mrs Lee was interviewed on her own, so it is not possible to know how her husband felt about the changing situation. But it was evident that she herself resented what she interpreted as her mother's possessiveness (see page 95) and said that, having been away from her mother for some time (Mrs Lee was an army wife), she felt that her mother was trying to make up for lost time.

These two cases illustrate a number of what are almost certainly general truths and also indicate something of how the age, sex, and marital status of carers are the products of complex social processes. In the first place, a certain change of status for the two daughters was taking place. Various degrees of resistance were being mounted to prevent these changes, not least from the daughters themselves; but other characters in the drama, with their own interests at heart, had also come forward to express their views and argue for the status quo. These characters were the husbands and the children of the daughters, and to a more limited extent other interested professionals such as their GPs. For example, according to Mrs Archer, her GP had advised her that she should on no account give up her full-time job – on the grounds, first, that he did not want another depressed and anxious patient on his hands and, secondly, that her father, whose doctor he also was, was suffering only from 'nerves'.

It is possible that once the negotiation appears to have had a 'conclusion', in the sense that someone has been identified as the primary carer, particularly if that person is a woman in some kind of kin relationship with the cared for, then that woman becomes identified as a 'carer' for ever and anon. This may explain why the other person caring for someone who still had a male spouse living was doing the amount of caring that she was – although see above (page 50) for Mrs Cook's own explanation as to why she was caring for her aunt. Mrs Cook was caring for her aunt as well as for her father. Her aunt's husband was still alive and apparently well. But long before her father and her aunt had become ill, Mrs Cook had taken on the role of carer. She had, three years before, nursed her terminally ill mother through the last stages of leukaemia, and at the end had moved into her parents' house for three months in order to provide full-time care fo her mother. No doubt this had been welcomed by her father, who was physically and mentally fit but aged 80 at the time. Once Mrs Cook had been identified – and identified herself – as primarily a carer, the exchange of one dependent elderly person for another seems to have been a relatively straightforward matter, and one that Mrs Cook accepted as part of the lot of being a daughter and a woman. Nevertheless, Mrs Cook's 'negotiated settlement' seemed to mean that the work she did for her father and her aunt should in no way interfere with the domestic services she provided for her husband. In order to fulfil her household 'duties' to three households, Mrs Cook rose at 5 a.m. and did not finish her own housework until around 10 p.m. When she had lived with her parents during the last stages of her mother's illness she had 'rushed home' every evening in order to get a meal for her husband and her son.

The cases of Mrs Archer and Mrs Lee indicate something of the process of becoming a carer and the way the age, sex, and marital status of carers are social products. In particular, where there is a 'choice' of carer between, on the one hand, an elderly and possibly incompetent man and, on the other hand, a relatively young woman who is *assumed* to be competent and with obligations deriving from kinship, then negotiations will come to a 'conclusion' once that woman has accepted her role as primary carer, in a way that is acceptable to her more immediate family of husband and children. Thereafter, once a carer, always a carer. Once that identity is fixed and agreed to by all the interested parties, it seems that elderly dependents can become relatively interchangeable. Mrs Cook dated her own caring for her father from the day her mother died; the additional caring for her aunt started a year later and was taken on in such a way that it did not disturb the arrangements for caring for either her father or her husband and son. This additional caring did not have to be renegotiated.

There was one respondent in the sample, however, who indicated how an apparent settlement could break down, particularly if a new factor was introduced into the situation or the original parties to the orginal settlement altered. Mr and Mrs Vaughan had, before moving to Canterbury, spent some time living with one or other of their two daughters, in the expectation that, should one of the elderly Vaughans die, the care of the other would automatically devolve upon one of these daughters. However, by the time of the interview, Mr Vaughan had once more become his wife's primary carer.

The Vaughans first decided that they had to move when Mr Vaughan first became seriously ill in 1978, and he felt he could no longer cope on his own with his wife's Parkinson's disease. His older daughter invited them to come and live with her and her husband, the idea being that Mr and Mrs Vaughan should continue to lead relatively separate lives in their own 'granny annexe'. As Mr Vaughan put it, this arrangement 'was a disaster from the word go'. An essential part of the 'settlement' – namely, the 'granny annexe' – almost immediately fell through because their daughter could not get the necessary planning permission. Moreover, almost immediately she was made redundant from her full-time job and decided to start her own business, running it from home. This would have meant that the Vaughans' daughter's home 'would have become like Piccadilly Circus'. The Vaughans decided that their five-month experiment in living with this daughter should be brought to a close. At this point their second daughter stepped into the breach and offered to buy, with her parents, a house already large enough to provide a 'granny annexe'. This new arrangement was welcomed by Mr and Mrs Vaughan, and they duly went to live with their younger daughter in what Mr Vaughan described as 'the ideal house'. Within three years, however, their son-in-law had left their daughter, and their daughter had found another man with whom she wanted to start a new life. All these changes meant that the original house had to be sold. Not only that: their daughter's new man wanted to move away from the Home Counties and did not want Mr and Mrs Vaughan to move with them. The 'ideal' arrangement was hastily brought to an end, and Mr and Mrs Vaughan were more or less left to their own devices. Almost as though the Vaughans were trying to dispel any ambiguity about who was caring for Mrs Vaughan, they had decided to move to Canterbury, a town where they knew no one and some considerable distance from both of their daughters. Although the elder daughter was, at the time of the interview, regularly visiting her parents once a week, it would have been impossible for her to see much more of them, let alone provide the kind of constant care they now needed.

Mr Vaughan had now negotiated a new settlement, not this time with his own kin, but with the professional social services, to whom he had written before moving to Canterbury. Such professionalized care, which is based not on the assumption of the continuity of affection but rather on the assumption of the continuity of 'need', might indeed prove more reliable and continuous than the informal and affection-based care available through the arangements made with kin.

Thus the case of the Vaughans demonstrates how, even where there seems to be a choice of carers between, on the one hand, one of two daughters and, on the other, an increasingly sick and elderly man, and where negotiations have taken place that seem to be satisfactory to all parties, the settlement can nevertheless founder when new factors are introduced into the situation. Perhaps the insistence on the 'granny annexe' was itself a symbolic and concrete recognition by all the parties involved that there were unresolved ambiguities left in these caring relationships between the parents and their daughters. These underlying ambiguities possibly made the caring relationships in question particularly vulnerable to changing circumstances.

Two more general points can be drawn out of these cases where the burden of care was in the process of being shifted from the elderly husband of an elderly wife to a woman in the younger generation. First, shifts in the burden of care from one generation to another can take place only if the generations remain geographically close to each other or else move towards each other. But, paradoxically, in cases where the generations already live close to each other, it is precisely because they are already within easy reach that ambiguities and tensions may continue over considerable periods of time. This is because no concrete decision about the division of labour between the two generations need take place until such time as a crisis occurs – when, for example, the elderly carer himself becomes ill and has to go into hospital. In these circumstances, shifts in the burden of care can be gradual and almost unnoticed, except by those most intimately involved. But such gradual evolution of new caring relationships, while appearing to be less disruptive in the sense that nobody has to move house, can also mean that the situation need never be properly discussed by the parties involved and that the evolution of new caring relationships may thus take place within an atmosphere of continuous tension and even considerable unhappiness. Where migration is a precondition of one generation taking over the burden of caring from another, at least one can expect that some discussion has taken place between the parties involved and some thought given to the implications. In other words, some kind of negotiated settlement is at least reached initially, and a general commitment to these new relationships made all round, even if, due to changing circumstances or the irritations of close proximity, such relationships founder at a later stage.

Secondly, I have suggested that where an elderly man is caring for his wife, the obligations of gendered kinship will cross-cut and contradict the obligations of marriage. In this sample, it was evident that the only caring relationships where there was some doubt as to who was actually 'the' carer were in situations of this kind. There is also some evidence from this small sample that, in a situation where an elderly woman is caring for her husband, she may be left to her own devices rather longer. In the first place, there were a number of caring relationships in this sample which seem to have started very abruptly when the person presently being cared for became a widow. Mrs Barnes, Mrs Evans, Mrs Green, and Mrs Hall all mentioned their mothers' or mothers-in-law's bereavement as a contextual reason as to why these elderly women had originally moved into their household or had come to live very close by. One can assume that these elderly women had been carers themselves, looking after their terminally ill husbands. It is also likely that the idea that these women carers were themselves in need of care had been post-poned until the demands on their caring services were over. For example, by the time Mrs Evans's mother and Mrs Barnes's mother-in-law were widowed they were already rather depen-dent. Mrs Evans's mother, who had cared for her father for twenty years, was practically blind and suffering from diabetes, while Mrs Barnes's mother-in-law was already showing signs of confusion when she returned from Spain, where she had cared for her husband until his death.

It would be a mistake to try to explain the number of caring relationships that started as a result of bereavement and widowhood purely in terms of the postponed need for care on the part of an elderly woman carer. Clearly there were other reasons at work; compassion for the lonely and sympathy for the bereaved were no doubt also strong enough motivations for some of these carers to ask their mothers or mothers-in-law to come and live with them. But, given what we know about the allocation of the formal helping services and the evidence from other studies that male carers seem more likely to receive some services, particularly home help (Bebbington and Davies 1983), it would be surprising if something of this pattern of the alloca-tion of the formal services were not echoed by (and echoing) the informal services, such that elderly women carers might be perceived by their own families to be better at coping than would an elderly man carer in similar circumstances. The cir-cumstances of three out of the four men carers in this sample go some way to confirm this view. All of them, except for Mr

Unwin, had no obvious alternative carer, since either they had no children or their children lived too far away to be of any help.

CONCLUSION

In this chapter I have suggested that, even if carers themselves claim that they were the 'obvious' carer in their particular situation, they are in important ways selected and self-selected. They are selected, first and foremost, according to dominant, normative, and gendered rules of kinship. It is in this sense, and only in this sense, that some of these carers in this sample could claim that their selection was 'obvious'. Secondly, they are selected according to how they and other members of their immediate nuclear family come to an agreement that caring is compatible with other demands on them from these family members. They are also self-selected. All these carers had chosen one particular form of care – informal care – over and above another form of care – formal care. In other words, they had chosen that their dependent kin should continue to live, as Miss Nicholson so succinctly put it, '*at* home rather than *in* a home'. In Chapters 4 and 5 we turn to the material and ideological context of that decision not to use residential care. Chapter 4 looks at the compatibility of caring with life-cycle and labour-market position, while Chapter 5 considers love and guilt as personal motivations to becoming a carer.

4
Reasons for caring: the material and life-cycle context

In Chapter 3 I described the kinship rules and the negotiation of the impact of those rules, according to which the carers in this sample had apparently been 'selected'. However, in the conclusion to that chapter I noted that these carers had also been 'self-selected'. By this I meant that, while one may describe the rules by which selection takes place, this does not wholly explain why a particular carer has put himself or herself forward for potential selection in the first place. In this chapter and Chapter 5 I shall argue that it is at that initial point in the selection process that some form of 'self-selection' takes place. Certain individuals, almost without exception (and for very important reasons) women, make a decision that, for particular elderly kin in their immediate kin network, they have a responsibility to ensure their care, and that care should be informal within a family setting, rather than formal within an institutional setting.

The basis on which this self-selection takes place is both material and ideological. By this I mean that there are certain material factors – in particular, position in the labour market, household resources, and the life-cycle of the carer – that encourage certain women to take up caring at particular points in their lives and to create a kind of 'mix' of caring with other demands on their time and their emotions; and there are also ideological factors, such as a dominant view that women should behave in a caring manner, a view which most women (and men) find irresistible. In this chapter I shall concentrate on the material factors that determine the selection of a carer and in Chapter 5 on the more ideological factors. It will not always be possible to stick to this somewhat crude dichotomy of the moti-vations to care; material factors are mediated by ideological factors, particularly when it comes to the selection, or self-selection, of women in the first place; and vice versa. Neverthe-less, the emphasis in each chapter is different. In this one we concentrate particularly on the life-cycle position of the carers, while in Chapter 5 we consider the reasons the carers them-selves gave for the caring they did, and especially their ideas of love and guilt.

The starting-point for this chapter is the data on the age, sex, and marital status of the carers and their cared for presented as *Tables 1* and *2* in Chapter 2. The analysis presented here began as an early attempt to make sense of those data, and to tease out the generalizations that might legitimately be made from such a small sample about the material foundation to the motivation to care. In the following discussion I shall first describe the life-cycle position of the men and women carers in the sample, and speculate as to why there were considerable differences be-tween the life-cycle positions of the male carers as opposed to those of the women carers interviewed. Second, I shall demon-strate that, in contrast to the men in the sample, the women had been in a wide variety of life-cycle positions at the point when they took up caring. In trying to explain why this variety of life-cycle positions seem to exist among women carers, I shall develop a life-cycle typology of caring which contains within it reference to women's position as mothers and their position as paid workers. Thirdly, as a continuous theme within the discus-sion, I shall attempt to use the life-cycle typology as a way of teasing out how far the women in this sample had 'volunteered' to care[1].

To recap, of the nineteen carers interviewed, fifteen were women, and four were men. All the men were caring for their wives, whereas eleven of the women were caring for someone

---

[1] The bulk of this chapter has been published elsewhere, entitled 'The Life Course and Informal Caring: Towards a Typology', in Cohen 1987.

other than their husband, usually a relative from the older generation. All the men carers were aged over 65, and one of them, at 84, was the oldest carer in the group. In contrast, as one would expect given that it was only the women who were caring for someone of a different generation from themselves, the women's ages spread over a much wider age range, with the youngest under 40 and the oldest in her late seventies. *Table 1* (page 35) summarizes the age and sex of the carers and cared for.

The considerable ages of the men carers, and more particularly the fact that all four of them were caring for their wives, as shown in *Table 2* (page 35), distinguished them from the women carers, the majority of whom were caring for someone other than their own spouse. It may well be that these age and marital status differences between the men and women carers have wider reference beyond this small sample, for they neatly illustrate a finding common to many other studies of caring (e.g. Nissel and Bonnerjea 1982). The point is that the men had taken on caring at a very different point in their life cycle from that of the women. All the men had been more or less retired when their wives had become incapable of looking after themselves or their husbands. It is highly unlikely, however, that had their wives become ill at an earlier stage in the life cycle, when these men were still in full-time paid work, they would have taken on full-time caring; almost certainly they would have found someone else (the Social Services Department, a daughter, a paid employee, or some combination of all three) to take it on, while they continued to earn enough to keep their wives and themselves in their accustomed environment. This suggestion is confirmed by the fact that three of these men held very traditional views about the position of women in society. Far from being unusually radical in their opinions, they had very strong ideas about the nature of the marriage relationship and the appropriate roles of men and women within it. For example, none of the wives of these three men had worked throughout their marriages, and their husbands described them as the kind of women who would never have wanted it otherwise. However, in the emergency circumstances they were now experiencing, these men were prepared to abandon completely the traditional domestic division of labour within marriage in order to maintain what they perceived to be the more important tradition of marriage itself (see Chapter 5).

Confirmation that men generally would be very reluctant, if not non-existent, carers at an earlier pre-retirement stage in their life cycles can be garnered from the experiences of four women in the sample who were caring for one of their husband's parents. All four women were married to husbands who were in full-time work. While one of the husbands, an academic, had taken to working at home rather more in order to keep his wife company while she cared for his mother, none of the other husbands had given up full-time work. Their wives had stepped into the breach. It would, as I have suggested above, be very unusual if they had given up work even to care for their wives. Many men (most?) would be likely to seek the aid of someone else to take over the caring task. This need not be simply a crude reflection of the prevailing sexual division of labour. For many men, particularly those in relatively well-paid and congenial work, a decision to remain in work, even if it means paying someone else to care for their wives, could be justified in terms not of the traditional sexual division of labour but of the maximization of household income at a time when household expenses, due to the illness of one of its members, are likely to be high.

Thus, as far as caring is concerned, I suggest that the male life cycle contains definite 'start-up' and 'cut-off' points oriented around paid work. Full-time paid work almost always acts as a buffer between the social and family circumstances of a man and his availability for caring. Once the period in the cycle of full-time paid work is over, a man suddenly becomes available for full-time caring. Indeed, the male life cycle is typically so full of these sudden changes in life-style and lifelong commitment that the prospect of taking up caring as a full-time retirement occupation probably appeals to some men, since their caring role can fill the time that may now hang heavily on their hands. Those retired men caring for their wives may also interpret such caring as reciprocity for the servicing their wives provided for them while well, and as a way of maintaining and justifying a lengthy marriage (see Chapter 5).

THE LIFE CYCLE OF WOMEN CARERS

In contrast to the men carers in the sample, the women carers were at a variety of positions in the life cycle both at the time of the interview and, as we shall see later, at the point in their lives when they took up caring.

As *Figure 1*, shows, in conjunction with *Table 1*, at the time of the interview the great majority of women carers (10 out of 15) were past the child-rearing, let alone child-bearing, stage. Of those who had had children (13 out of the 15) only 5 still had a child or children living permanently at home. It will be seen that only 2 women were still mothering children under 15 years of age, and the remaining 3 women fully expected their children to leave home to enter further or higher education very shortly. None of these five women expected their children to stay at home beyond the age of 18 to 19. They could all put a time limit to the period they would have to provide a steadily decreasing amount of care for their children; their problem was that none of them could put a time limit to the period over which they would have to care for an increasingly dependent elderly person. Thus, just as they were reaching the point in the life cycle where most women would expect to be able to make somewhat self-indulgent plans for their own future, these women were facing an indefinite period of caring.

However, *Figure 1* represents a 'snapshot' taken at the time of interview. In *Figure 2* I have crudely calculated the ages of the youngest children at the moment when the married women carers with children actually started caring. Such a diagram-matic representation necessarily simplifies the complicated pro-cess of becoming a carer by giving the start of caring a definite date; nevertheless, the figure does show that the life-cycle position was rather different and that, at the time they began the tasks of caring, rather more of these married women were re-sponsible for school-age children (and, in two cases, babies) than they were by the time of interview. The most important point made by *Figure 2* is that, for many of these women, the initiation of caring for an elderly dependent person *coincided* with child care. Thus, far from indicating (as *Figure 1* does) an idea of entrapment and frustrated ambitions, *Figure 2* suggests a willingness – indeed, a positive choice – to care, at a point in the

Figure 1 Number of women carers, at the time of interview, by age of youngest child living at home, by whether or not woman carer in paid work

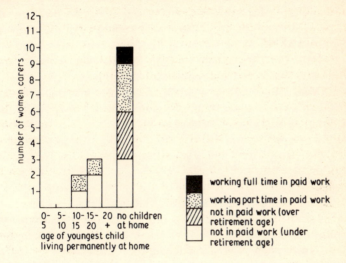

Figure 2 Number of married women carers with children, by age of youngest child at 'start' of caring

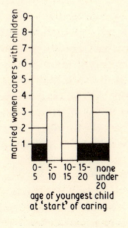

life cycle when many of these women were already engaged in caring for their healthy but quite young children.

In the following paragraphs I shall attempt to set up a typology of women's motivation to care, using life-cycle position and employment prospects as the crucial variables. In the analysis I shall exclude the four women carers who were caring for their husbands and concentrate only on those eleven women carers who were caring across generations. This is on the grounds that, given that I am positing a choice to care, the marriage relationship contains so many coercive elements as to largely exclude options, at least in the short run.

I   WOMEN WHO TAKE ON CARING WHILE THEIR CHILDREN ARE STILL AT HOME

As *Figure 2* shows, five out of the eleven married women carers under consideration started caring when their children were under the age of 15 and still at school. One woman (Mrs Knowles) started caring for her mother – in the sense that her mother moved into a 'granny annexe' in their house – when she was pregnant with her youngest child. Why did these women take on these additional caring tasks in such a way that they coincided with child care?

(a) Reciprocal exchange of services

It is frequently argued by commentators (Bulmer 1986) that caring relationships can be satisfactorily founded on some notion of the reciprocal exchange of services. If that is the case, then there seem to me to be two problems about reciprocity across generations. First, the exchange of services can have very long time-lags. Elderly people may be able to make some contribution to the care of infants and very small children, but as they grow more frail they will be less and less able to provide such assistance and they themselves will increasingly be in need of care.

Secondly, the provision of caring services for children has a time limit to it. Children eventually become less dependent, and at certain crucial ages they start to leave home to go first to school and perhaps college and then (hopefully) to work. The provision of caring services for old people has no such time limit, nor such obvious landmarks of reductions in dependency. Thus services rendered to old people may stretch over a very much longer period than services to children.

Nevertheless, despite these problems, there seems little doubt that some carers do at least start off with some idea of potential reciprocity between carer and cared for. This seems to have been the case with Mrs Knowles. When Mrs Knowles's mother came to live with them in a 'granny annexe', despite the fact that both Mr and Mrs Knowles had regarded the arrival of this 66-year-old lady with some trepidation, they had nevertheless hoped that she would be able to help out with the care of the young family. This she did in fact do. That was thirteen years before the interview. Since then the reciprocal services between mother and daughter had grown more and more unequal, partly because the need for help with child care was no longer so pressing, but also because Mrs Knowles's mother was increasingly disabled. Mrs Knowles (who was 47) was one of the few women in this sample who was clearly now straining at the leash to get out into the labour market – something, she said a little wistfully, she hoped to be able to do 'before I reach retirement age!' Thus this case seems to illustrate the possibility that the *idea* of reciprocity may initiate a caring relationship, particularly when a carer's children are infants and hence relatively easy to handle. But the *practice* of reciprocity becomes very diluted and increasingly one-sided as the caring relationship continues, such that other feelings like resentment and frustration come to obscure it and even eclipse it altogether.

(b) Construction of elderly person as another infant

It is possible that some women will volunteer to care for an elderly dependent person when they have very young children at home on the grounds that the old person can be relatively easily absorbed into the already existing daily round of domestic and caring services. In other words, the elderly person can be 'reconstructed' as an infant – at least in terms of the time and services that have to be expended in his or her care, if not in terms of personality. Within this sample there was no woman who fitted this description exactly, although one woman showed that the reconstruction of an adult dependant into another infant may be one way of handling what would otherwise be a catastrophe. This was Mrs Fisher, one of the four married women whom I have excluded from this general discussion. But it is worth mentioning her to point out that the onset of her husband's dependency, as a result of a brain haemorrhage when her son was only a year old, meant that she became in effect the mother of two 'infants' and the head of a single-parent family. Her disappointment at this terrible turn of events must have been very nearly overwhelming, but the fact that she was already at home caring for one infant may have made it easier for her to take on the care of an additional person. (However, there are no doubt many other women who would claim, with legitimacy, that the care of an infant precludes the care of an additional dependent adult.)

(c) As children reach school age – caring as a legitimate alternative to paid work

Increasingly in Britain, as women reach the stage in their lives when they are no longer needed at home to care for pre-school-age children, they take up part-time work. In 1981, 57 per cent of women whose youngest child was over 5 but under 16 were economically active; and of those women, the large majority were in part-time work (OPCS 1984: tables 4–6). The contribution of the wife's earnings to the household resources is often crucial, and women with school-age children who do not have paid work of any kind are an increasingly small minority. Some of these women may be unable, rather than unwilling, to find work due to the present high levels of unemployment; others, however, may for whatever reason prefer not to work, particularly those women living in households where the resources are already more than adequate for the standard of living they and their families want. Many women who married in the 1950s and the early 1960s gave up work, not on the birth of the first child, but on *marriage*. Both they and their husbands are likely still to be strongly committed to the idea that women should not work even when their children are old enough to look after themselves, at least for part of the day.

For such women, with children at school and an adequate

standard of living, time may well hang heavy on their hands. A number of factors prevent them from taking up paid work, notably the attitudes of their own husbands and the fact that they may not have the skills necessary for work that would be congruent with the social standing they have acquired through their husbands' employment and place in the community. A 'career' as a carer does not disturb their own, their husband's, or their community's image of who and what they are.

In this sample, there was one woman who demonstrated some of these characteristics. Mrs Barnes had given up work as a fully qualified SRN when she had married Mr Barnes (a prominent local business man) in 1964. She had not worked since, despite the fact that her own children were now in the sixth form and at school-leaving age. Mrs Barnes thought of the unpaid caring work she did as very like the paid work she used to do; her use of language made this very clear:

'I left work when I married. But since then it's been quite incredible how one's "on call" so often for people. I've had lots of "patients" since! . . . It's definitely true that I'm more willing to care for Gran because I'm a nurse. And because I'm a nurse I can look at it as just another job.'

As a result of her mother-in-law's increasing dependency, Mrs Barnes had given up a number of voluntary and community-oriented activities (such as active participation in the Nurses' League and what she called 'my rugby teas for the school') and replaced these activities with other outside activities largely oriented around caring, including being a founder member of the Carers' Support Group and serving on its committee. At no point in the interview did Mrs Barnes indicate that she missed paid work or that she had any intention of returning to it. At the end of the interview she turned to me as I was leaving and said, 'I just don't know *what* I'll do when Gran goes.'

Thus the case of Mrs Barnes indicates that, particularly at certain points in the class structure, custom and resources simultaneously operate to keep certain women out of the labour market even when they have reached the point in their personal life cycle when they have the time and the interest to take on some kind of paid work. They are 'career' carers. Such women constitute a no doubt diminishing pool of domestic labour to whom the opportunity to care for someone might actually come as something of a relief, as a way of avoiding what might otherwise take on the dimensions of a domestic crisis.

I suggest that this is a diminishing pool of unpaid labour for two reasons. First, the number of women who do not expect to combine paid work with marriage at some point in their life cycle must by now be very small (Martin and Roberts 1984: ch. 12). Secondly, the number of married couples with dependent children who can nevertheless afford to remain a single-earner household must also be diminishing.

(d) As children reach school age – caring in addition to paid work

If women in paid employment take on caring they will be subject to three sets of demands on their time: their husbands and children, their paid work, and the care of the elderly relative. One might expect such women to illustrate a number of themes. First, the demands on their time are such that one might expect many women to avoid the tasks of caring if they possibly can, and for those who do agree to it to be exceptional along some identifiable dimension. Secondly, one might expect the contribution that such women make to the household finances to be fairly considerable – not necessarily in terms of absolute amounts but in proportionate terms to the total amount of household income. If that is the case then two things would follow: first, they would be reluctant to give up work or reduce their hours in spite of the enormous stresses on their time; but, secondly, they may be willing to give up work altogether or reduce their hours as their children grow into financial independence. Thirdly, it would be surprising if such women were in paid employment that in any sense constituted a 'career'. Given the other demands on their time, their part-time work would have to be of the kind that makes few emotional and motivational demands. It may also be the case that their husbands are in employment that is either not particularly well paid or somewhat insecure, thus making it all the more important for their wives to remain in work despite other considerable calls on their time.

In this sample, two women (Mrs Cook and Mrs Lee) were continuing to work part-time while caring for an elderly relative and had also been, at least when they began caring, responsible for the care of school-age children. Similarly, Mrs Evans, who had been caring for her mother for twenty-six years, had been in part-time work and looking after a 6-year-old when her mother first came to live with her and her family. All three women demonstrated some of the characteristics that I suggest above might distinguish such women who willingly take on caring despite already existing calls on their time. First, all of them made it clear to me that they thought there were special reasons why, when they first realized that their mothers needed special care, they were the only people in their immediate kin network who could possibly take on that responsibility. Mrs Lee was an only child. Mrs Cook was not an only child but was an only daughter – a social fact to which she herself accorded some significance (see page 93). Mrs Evans had been in a somewhat similar position although, in her case, she had two siblings, a brother and a sister. Mrs Evans's brother's wife had always made it clear that she had no intention of having Mrs Evans's mother – not even to give Mr and Mrs Evans a holiday. Mrs Evans's sister had emigrated after the war (see page 43).

Thus these three women shared one significant special characteristic. It so happened that the people they were caring for when they began caring became highly dependent just at the point in the life cycle when these women had been relieved of the care of a pre-school-aged child and had also taken on part-time work. In all three cases there seems to have been a genuine crisis of dependency. Mrs Lee's mother had a very severe heart attack; Mrs Cook's mother was diagnosed as having leukaemia; and Mrs Evans's mother was recently bereaved, and her sight was failing fast. Moreover, at the time when these crises occurred there seemed (at least to them) to be no one else in their immediate kin network who could do the work. Certain elements of *chance* (mediated by sex-role ideology) combined to ensure that these particular women felt under considerable pressure to take on caring, even though their time was already heavily committed elsewhere.

None of the three women had, at the time they started caring, been on a 'career' ladder of employment. Mrs Lee had so far found that caring for her mother fitted in with her morning working hours, since she could visit her parents in the afternoons before her children came home from school. However, both Mrs Cook and Mrs Evans had to make changes to their working hours, and Mrs Evans had eventually and much to her regret given up work altogether.

Unfortunately, it is impossible to confirm whether these three women made proportionately large contributions to their households' resources as a result of their paid work, and hence whether pressures of financial need largely motivated their willingness to spread their time in three different directions. Certainly none of the three women had husbands in particularly well-paid employment. Among this tiny and unrepresentative sample their household income was probably lower than average.

I have argued, then, that some women will take on caring even though their time is already heavily committed in both paid and unpaid work when basically three conditions hold. First, a fortuitous set of circumstances whereby an elderly person becomes ill combines with another set of circumstances whereby the carer feels that she and only she is available to care for the elderly person. (I emphasize the word 'she' because it is important to bear in mind that no man already active in the labour market is likely to regard himself – or be regarded – as the carer of the last resort in the same way as a woman would.) Secondly, the carer is not engaged in a 'career' to which she wants to devote herself body and soul and is highly likely to be in part-time rather than full-time work. However, thirdly, the proportionate contribution that the carer makes to the household income is likely to be relatively high, such that the household would be in financial difficulty if she gave up paid work. Finally, let us remember that some women carers will simply refuse to give up paid work even if it causes enormous strains on their time because it is only at work that they derive some status other than that of a domestic and unpaid worker in the home. Of the three women discussed in this section, Mrs Evans made it clear that she regretted giving up work to care for her mother because she had been lonely ever since. For every Mrs Evans who gives up work there are probably many other women carers who continue to work part-time because they regard their work as crucial to their sense of self.

II WOMEN WHO TAKE ON CARING AS THEIR CHILDREN ARE LEAVING HOME OR LONG AFTER THEIR CHILDREN HAVE LEFT HOME

(a) To prevent the 'empty nest' syndrome

By the time the children are about to leave or have left home, one can expect that in the 1980s most of their mothers will be in their late forties to early fifties. Before their marriage most of these women will have worked, although very few of them will have left the parental home to do so. After marriage, although most of them will have continued to work until the birth of their first child, between a quarter and a third of them will have given up work on marriage (Martin and Roberts 1984).

The older these women are the less likely they are to have returned to work after the birth of their first child and the longer the time taken to return to work after the last birth (Martin and Roberts 1984: ch. 9). Nevertheless, paid work is important to women of all ages; indeed, Martin and Roberts suggest that, by the time women at present aged 50 to 59 are 60, they will have spent 59 per cent of their possible working time at work (1984: table 9.5). Yet it is also true that women at present over the age of 50 have, over their recent past, been rather more child-care-oriented than work-oriented relative to younger cohorts of women.

Mrs Jackson, the wife of an academic, had had four children and was now caring for her mother-in-law. At the time her mother-in-law came to live with the Jacksons they had two children aged 15 and 17 still living at home; the older two had already left home. A few years earlier, seeing that her children were well on the way to independence, Mrs Jackson had decided to retrain as a teacher and subsequently got a part-time job as a schoolteacher. However, Mrs Jackson discovered she was not altogether happy with her job, and when after a few years she also found that she would need some time off from the school in order to recover from an operation, she decided to resign. It was at this juncture, with her children rapidly growing up and away, that her mother-in-law became seriously ill at the age of 87 and had to spend some time in hospital. On the discharge of the old lady, Mrs Jackson volunteered to care for her even though others seemed to be available to take on the task (see page 48). Mrs Jackson therefore was both voluntarily prolonging her caring responsibilities and thereby postponing what might otherwise have been a rather painful period in her life. It seems that the moment when the old lady became in need of care coincided with a patch in Mrs Jackson's life when she was looking around for someone to care for, at least in the short run, while she once again rethought her future. With the end of motherhood staring her in the face, her mother-in-law must have appeared as something of a *dea ex machina*.

There are certain parallels between Mrs Jackson and Mrs Barnes, whom I have previously described as a 'career' carer, and, as we shall see in the next section, with Mrs Green. Both Mrs Jackson and Mrs Barnes had husbands in well-paid work, and their own potential contribution from any paid work they might do was not essential for the financial survival of the household. If paid work was not necessary for the income it generated, then, for different reasons, neither did it hold out many other attractions. Both women had taken on unpaid caring in order to avoid or postpone paid work and to prolong domesticity.

Such women cannot be that unusual. As I have suggested, there is something of a cohort of women who married in the 1950s and early 1960s for whom prolonged domesticity may still conform with their more youthful intentions. There are, however, almost certainly class dimensions that determine who, within this cohort, will now be available for caring, since the decision to care necessarily entails taking on the extra expense of caring for someone at the same time as rejecting the possibility of becoming a two-earner household. Such class dimensions may also coincide with tenure and age dimensions, since, if the household is in owner-occupation *and* the mortgage is paid off, then such households will not only have lost the expense of caring for children but also have, by the time the couple have reached their middle fifties, very considerably reduced housing costs. In contrast, council tenants, whose housing costs tend to rise with inflation and come down only when household income is drastically reduced through retirement, would not be as freely available; almost certainly they would have to combine caring with some form of employment for the female carer.

To talk in terms of the special characteristic of a particular age cohort indicates that women in future will be less willing to postpone or avoid paid work when their children grow up and away. That may be the case, although there are also countervailing tendencies, one predictable, the other less so. In the first place, given the expansion of owner-occupation in recent years, it will increasingly be the case that many households will find that their children have left home just at the point when their housing costs are also drastically reduced. Thus, in financial terms, there will be fewer households who find themselves in the position of having to have two earners in order to maintain the standard of living that they have come to expect in their middle age. If that is the case, it may also follow that women in younger age cohorts will be willing to make themselves available for caring at this point in the life cycle. Secondly, the prospects for employment of both men and women are unpredictable; it may be that by the time the cohorts of women at present bearing and rearing small children reach their own middle age, the availability of paid work for them will be somewhat reduced, and they would in principle be available for caring. On the other hand, it is possible that men's unemployment will be higher than women's, particularly in some parts of the country, in which case more women will have to go out to work in order for the household simply to survive. Whether unemployed men will take on the tasks of caring is a moot point; the research on domestic labour and paid work rather indicates that they will not (Pahl 1984).

(b) Caring as a legitimate alternative to paid work: the importance of health

As the case of Mrs Jackson above makes clear, there are some women who take up caring because they think they will prefer it to paid work. But there was at least one other woman in the sample who had taken up caring in order to be able legitimately to give up paid work. Mrs Green was married to a local-government officer and had, until recently, worked as a cashier/book-keeper in a multiple store. She told me that she gave up work because 'I could see this coming.' Although, at the time she gave up work, none of her elderly relatives were in immediate need of care, Mrs Green fully expected that her services could be called upon at any time. This was because she seemed to be the only woman in the immediate kin network of both her parents-in-law and her mother, since both Mr and Mrs Green had been only children.

Mrs Green's resignation from work had also coincided with a period of illness from which she knew she would need some time to recover. This seems to me to be rather important, especially because a similar story emerged from Mrs Jackson. Given that many women in their fifties do experience quite severe health problems they may think that they will find caring less of a strain on their health than paid work. However, giving up work in favour of unpaid caring on health grounds may not be entirely voluntary. With so many women in *part-time* paid work, their rights to remain in a job, especially those employed less than sixteen hours a week, are not fully protected under the employment protection legislation. They are neither protected from dismissal, should they need to take time off work over a long period on grounds of sickness, nor eligible for sick-pay under the National Insurance scheme. Moreover, even if they are eligible under that scheme, the fact that employers are now responsible for the first six weeks of sick-pay with time-lags in repayment from central government means that there are also considerable incentives on employers to dismiss their eligible employees if they possibly can. Thus women in their middle fifties who become ill are particularly vulnerable to 'persuasion' or even 'enforcement' to leave their jobs altogether, just at the point in their life cycle when they are likely to have elderly kin becoming increasingly frail. Assuming that their husbands continue to work until the men's retirement age of 65, these women will have approximately fifteen years in which they have nothing to do but keep a largely empty house. The opportunity to care for an elderly relative may indeed appear as something of a godsend since it both legitimizes their apparent 'idleness', provides an occupation for their time, and may also, at least initially, offer some companionship in what would otherwise be a rather isolated and potentially boring life.

But before leaping to the conclusion that illness in middle age drives many women to caring we should also remember that, just as with women who take on caring to postpone the 'empty

nest syndrome', so there may well be class and income dimensions to these women's willingness to care. Morbidity is not a
fixed or finite state, and it is highly likely that many middle-aged
women who need the money for themselves and their households will continue to struggle into paid work when their bodies
are crying out in protest and against their own (and others')
better judgement.

(c) Caring in addition to paid work

Mrs Jackson and Mrs Green, both of whom had ostensibly given
up work to care for an elderly relative, were somewhat unusual
women. Most women continue to work even when they have an
elderly relative to care for. According to Martin and Roberts,
among women up to age 59 who were caring for an elderly
relative, 58 per cent were still economically active, of whom just
over half were working part-time (Martin and Roberts 1984:
table 8.35). Unfortunately, Martin and Roberts do not break
their employment and caring data down by age or life-cycle
stage; but given that they also found that in their sample of
women aged up to 59 the majority of carers (70 per cent) were
over 40 years old (1984: table 8.91), we have to assume that the
majority of women in their sample who were caring but whose
children had left home were still in paid work of some kind. In
section Id, where the women who had remained in work at the
time they took on caring despite also having quite young children were under discussion, I suggested that these women
probably stayed in work because they and their families particularly needed their financial contribution and also because their
paid work was important to them as a source of independence
and sense of self. And in section IIb I said that there may be
rather special reasons why women without the care of children
give up paid work apparently in order to care for an elderly
person. Those reasons, I argued, probably have a considerable
amount to do with their own health, their attitude towards their
health and paid work, and their rights to remain in a particular
job despite needing a long period of convalescence.

However, most women in their fifties are in active and
good health and, even if they are not, they continue to work.
Thus it would have been extremely surprising if, even in this

unrepresentative sample, there were not some women who continued to work, especially among those women whose children had left home.

There were, in fact, two women who had no children living at home at the time they started caring and who were still in paid work at the time of the interview. These were Mrs Hall and Miss Nicholson, who had one significant thing in common. Both of them had organized their lives in such a way that of all the carers they, and one other, were the ones who had sufficiently extensive help to suggest that they should be considered 'joint' carers with one other person without whom it would have been out of the question for either of them to continue in paid work (see pages 38–40). Both of them had particularly pressing reasons for wanting to stay in paid work. In Miss Nicholson's case her determination probably reflected the fact that she particularly needed that continuity in her life in order to maintain her self-identity. In Mrs Hall's case it is interesting that she struggled into work despite being quite severely disabled with arthritis. Indeed, her 'joint' caring arrangement had really got going only when she had had to go into hospital for an operation on her knee and she had decided that, rather than leave her mother entirely in her husband's care, she needed the further help of her friend and neighbour. Her household depended on her earnings from her thirty-hours-a-week job, and in recently purchasing their council house they had incurred a considerable debt at an age when most owner-occupiers would be about to finish paying their mortgage. Although I have no hard-and-fast data to indicate as much, I suspect that the Halls were in no position to become a single-earner household with the additional expense of caring for Mrs Hall's mother.

Having suggested that both these carers were completely dependent on the services of the 'joint' carer in their lives to allow them to continue in paid work, the corollary to this arrangement is also important; if either of these 'joint' caring arrangements breaks down, then neither of these carers will be able to carry on working. A parallel situation exists for those women carers who first take on caring while they are still in paid work and are unable to find someone else with whom to share the caring work. For them there must eventually come a point when the needs of the person they are caring for are such that they feel they can no longer remain in paid work and have to give it up in order to care for their dependant full-time. In this sample two women had found themselves in that position; Mrs Mitchell had given up work to care for her husband, and Mrs Evans had eventually and reluctantly given up work to care for her mother.

CONCLUSIONS

In this chapter I began by distinguishing between the life cycles of the men and women carers in this sample and suggested that the importance of full-time paid work in men's life cycles was enough to 'blot out' any other calls upon their time. Women, on the other hand, experience life as a conglomeration of continuous demands emanating from different sources. Hence it is not surprising that the women carers in this sample started caring at a variety of points in their personal life cycles. This is not to say that the other demands on women's time, namely child care and paid work, are not important in determining whether or not, at a particular point in her life, a woman will become available or decide to become available for the caring task. But a woman will, if possible, combine these roles of mother, paid worker, and carer or, at the very least, juggle them together in order to maximize the servicing that she can adequately provide for members of her family.

At the start of the discussion of the life-cycle position of women carers, I distinguished between the women carers' life-cycle position at the time of the interview with their position at the time when they began caring. In so doing two things became clear. First, the women carers may well have been feeling particularly frustrated with their caring at the time of the interview, since almost all of them had finished caring for their children or were well within sight of that goal, and hence caring was increasingly incongruent with the rest of their lives. But secondly, by looking at the stage in the life cycle when these women took on caring it was possible to see that some had initiated caring at a point in their lives when the tasks of caring were particularly compatible with other domestic parts of their lives. For this reason, where caring occurs between generations rather than between spouses, it appears to fit in with particular life-cycle stages, and there seems to be an element of 'voluntariness' about the initiation of the caring relationship. Given the other two calls on women's time – namely, child care and paid work – I suggest that these two factors might be the crucial variables in analysing the decision to care.

Ideally, an analysis of the decision to care should include an analysis of the decision not to care. If that were possible then one might see more clearly how far some people do 'volunteer' to care and what are the particular circumstances under which they make that decision. But in a study of carers only, the best one can do is look at the particular variables that may affect that decision and how far those variables seem to tell a sensible and internally consistent story. It is this largely inductive method that I have used to draw up a typology of the decision by women to take on caring for someone other than their husbands. In that typology I assumed that life-cycle position and position in the labour market (both actual and potential) were crucial variables and have analysed the interviews within that framework. For that typology I devised the following categories.

Women with children
at the initiation of caring
(a) Reciprocity of care
(b) Construction of elderly
    person as another infant   } pre-school children

(c) Caring as a legitimate
    alternative to paid work
(d) Caring in addition to
    paid work   } school-age children

Women without children
at the initiation of caring
(a) To prevent the 'empty
    nest' syndrome'
(b) Caring as a legitimate
    alternative to paid work:
    the importance of health
(c) Caring in addition to paid
    work

↓

Pressure to give up paid work

For each category in this typology I discussed cases that seemed to demonstrate some of the reasons why women, at those particular points in their lives, should apparently 'choose' to take on caring.

I am certain this typology is not complete. For one thing, it has taken account of the circumstances only of married and never-married women and excludes the circumstances of divorced and separated women simply because they did not occur in this small sample. This typology is only an interpretation of the circumstances of the women carers whom I interviewed, and should be treated as a research tool rather than as a research finding. There is one more extremely important proviso to make about it. I have referred throughout this particular discussion to the element of 'voluntariness' in the motivation to care; but this is to lose the sense in which *no* woman is a 'volunteer'. By this I mean that women, in contrast to men, are subject to considerable ideological and material pressure to be the carers of the last resort, largely irrespective of their personal circumstances and of whether or not as individuals they would rather spend their time in paid work or caring more completely for their children (see Chapters 3 and 5). In this sample there was not a single man who was caring for someone other than his wife; moreover, all these caring men had started caring after retirement. In other words, only women are apparently the appropriate people to combine caring with paid work and child care and to care for dependants of a different generation from themselves. But within the general group of women as a whole there is usually some choice as to which particular woman should take on caring when it is called for. There were at least some women in this sample who did not seem to be the most obvious candidates to care for the particular elderly person for whom they had assumed responsibility. Some of the reasons why they apparently 'volunteered' have been outlined in the discussion in this chapter and in Chapter 3; other reasons, more concerned with individual feelings than with labour-market position or life-cycle point, will be discussed in Chapter 5.

There are both considerable parallels and interesting contrasts between the care of elderly dependants and the care of children. In the first place, neither the care of small children nor the care of elderly dependants is compatible with full-time work unless some alternative form of supplementary care can be found from within the kin or marital network, from the public sector or from private sources. But pressures to work and the availability of time to work increase as children grow older, while, in contrast, as the elderly age even further, there are considerable pressures on the carer to reduce working hours or to give up work altogether. However, just as with child care, the care of the elderly and women's position in the labour market are inextricably linked. Lower wages and lack of protection for periods off work, linked to part-time working, all combine to make women rather than men the likely carers should it become necessary to care for a relative at home. Similarly caring may in itself weaken women's labour-market position because of the need to take time off work when crises occur. Where women expect to have to take on the full-time care of an elderly person at some time in the future, this may well stop those women from pursuing goals related to their position in the labour market.

Caring for an elderly dependant is nevertheless *unlike* child care in one important respect. Children have only one mother; elderly people generally have more than one child or child-in-law. In other words, the network of obligations and pressures on mothers to care for their children is rather different from the comparable pressures on children to care for their parents or parents-in-law. Mothers are spotlighted. Children, and especially daughters and daughters-in-law, are simply lit; their position in their personal life cycle provides the stage backdrop.

5
Reasons for caring: love and duty

In Chapter 4 I outlined a typology which might cover the material basis to the motivation to care. I suggested that position in the life cycle and, for women, the compatibility of caring with other parts of their lives, particularly paid work and the unpaid work of child care, might deeply influence their initial motivation to care.

There is little doubt in my mind that the carers interviewed in this study would object strongly to this material formulation of their motivation. Chapter 4 relied heavily on my own interpretation of the material events and factors in their lives; that chapter's very dryness reflects the fact that the people interviewed themselves hardly referred to material factors, except to point out if they had found that caring interfered with paid work, or to mention the cost of caring and the adequacy – or otherwise – of the attendance allowance. Their own explanations of their motivation, and the language they used to tell me why they did the caring work they did, were couched in terms of personal feeling: love, guilt, compassion for another human being, gratitude for the one-time love and care of a now incapacitated mother or wife. It seems to me that these two rather different ways of explaining motivation are not incompatible; to some extent the two sets of explanation refer to the somewhat cliché-ridden duality of materialism and ideology. But to say that Chapter 4 was largely concerned with material motivation, and that the present chapter is largely concerned with ideology, would be to deny the strength of compassion and real love that many of these carers felt for the person for whom they were caring. Despite this chapter's emphasis on the ideological dimension to motivation, particularly in the discussion of guilt, some at least of the carers felt a strong loving basis to the caring they did. Let us now consider the language they used and their expressions of feeling.

MEN'S LOVE, WOMEN'S DUTY

As has been indicated, all the male carers were caring for their spouses, while eleven of the fifteen women carers were caring for their parents or parents-in-law. This difference was in itself probably a major part of the explanation for the sex differences that emerged between the men and women carers when they came to talk about the reasons why they were caring. For, on the whole, the men used the language regarded as the language of marriage – that of love – while the women, even in two cases the women caring for their husbands, used the language of duty.

Of the four men carers, three were at pains to impress upon me throughout the interview that the reason they were caring for their wives was that they cared *about* them. As Mr Vaughan said, in answer to the question as to why he helped his wife in the way that he did:

'I love her – it's as simple as that! I promised at my wedding; I meant the vows at the time and will always mean them.'

Similarly, Mr Young said, in answer to the same question, 'It's according to the marriage vows – and I love the girl, I suppose.'

Mr Williams said, 'It's the most natural thing in the world to do; she's my wife!'

While all these quotes indicate that the men felt that marriage had in itself obligated them to take on the caring task, they nevertheless took every possible opportunity to tell me that they also loved their wives dearly. Mr Young said that the aspect of caring that gave him the most satisfaction was 'to see her old eyes light up – oh, she's beautiful. Lovely natured, too.'

Mr Vaughan said, 'I love her dearly. I feel intensely sorry for her. I can't do enough to help her.'

And Mr Williams set his love for his wife within the context of the history of their long and difficult courtship:

'My wife came to me against the wishes of her family. It was a very special relationship, and I was determined that she should not regret it. She's a wonderful wife.'

The one male carer who did not express this kind of feeling for his wife was the one who, on the very day of the interview, had determined to have his wife admitted permanently to the local mental hospital. Mr Unwin was the only working-class man in the sample, and on retirement from his job at the local bakery he and his wife had begun to have considerable money problems. He explained that five years before, when 'the old age pension wasn't so kind to us as it is now', he and his wife were 'getting on each other's nerves'. Mr Unwin dated the inception of his wife's senile dementia to this period; he seemed to blame himself for some of her illness and, in particular, the aggression she continuously expressed towards him. Mr Unwin was also the only male carer whose wife had been diagnosed as suffering from senile dementia and he found it difficult to handle the particular form of aggression that often characterizes the early stages of that disease. Also, unlike the other men carers in the sample, Mr Unwin was getting no Social Services help at all. Thus, in Mr and Mrs Unwin's relationship there was little space left for the kind of love that the other male carers claimed underlay their determination to continue their marriages. While Mr Unwin clearly felt considerable *concern* for his wife, he nevertheless also felt that they would both be better off if their marriage came to a *de facto* end.

By distinguishing the claimed motivation of the men carers from that of their female counterparts, I have, by implication, indicated that the women carers used a different language and expressed different motivations for the caring that they did. As I will argue later, there *were* generalizable differences between how the men and the women carers talked about their personal motivation, but it would nevertheless be mistaken to assume that *none* of the women used the language of love. Some of the women did explain their motivation at least partially in terms of love, although, as we shall see, this was often with reference to their feelings in the past rather than the present.

Before turning to a general discussion of the motivation of the women carers, it is useful to compare with the men carers the motivation of that group of women carers whose caring relationship was most like that of the men – namely, the four women who were caring for their husbands. All of these four women were in themselves slightly atypical, although within the group of four they shared some important characteristics. Two of them had been caring for very long periods indeed; Mrs Osborne had cared for her husband for forty-one years, and Mrs Fisher for twenty-nine years. (No other carer in the sample, male or female, had been caring for more than twenty years, and most had been caring for considerably less than ten years.) Similarly, the two other women in this group of four shared another significant characteristic, one which they both referred to when they explained their commitment to caring; Mrs Mitchell and Mrs Ingram were both practising Catholics. (While a few other carers did refer to norms and obligations based on their religious beliefs, none of the others were so explicit as Mrs Mitchell and Mrs Ingram about the importance of their religion both as a motivation and as a potential source of comfort.)

Of these four women caring for their husbands, two used the language of love in an unqualified way to explain what they were doing. For Mrs Osborne there seemed to be no alternative, she had met her husband when she was a nurse and he was in hospital recovering from polio, and she had married him knowing that he would be permanently and severely disabled. Mrs Osborne said that neither of them had been 'spring chickens' when they had married (he had been 40 and she 35), and she had known what she was doing. Mr Osborne, who was present throughout the interview with his wife, described her as being 'very brave' to marry him. In other words, *as a result* of the onset of love, Mrs Osborne had become a carer. Mr Osborne's special needs had always been part and parcel of their marriage relationship, and for this reason there was an unspoken assumption that love had been the major motivating factor for Mrs Osborne since the relationship had begun. Mrs Osborne strongly objected to being called a 'carer', claiming instead that she was merely behaving as a wife.

Mrs Fisher also talked of her husband, who had had a very severe brain haemorrhage twenty-nine years before when their only son was less than a year old, with love and affection. She said, 'I love him so much, I won't let him be taken away.' When asked how she and her husband had got along together before he became ill, she said, 'Oh fine. We were very happy. We still are.' But Mrs Fisher's feelings about her husband and how her life had been affected by his long illness were also somewhat mixed:

'I think: I've got him and thank God. But sometimes I've wondered if I prayed too hard for him to live.'

Later in the interview she revealed how she believed that God had saved her husband and therefore given her the strength to care for him:

'I'm sure God is with me. I say my prayers every night. I'm a firm believer. I prayed so hard that He would spare him when he was ill and I'm sure He gives me the strength to do what I do.'

Mrs Fisher's discussion of her motivation referred not only to her love for her husband and her belief in God's support. In order to explain why she did what she did she also used a word that almost all the other women carers used to explain their motivation. When I asked Mrs Fisher whether she could think what it was that made her help her husband, she said:

'No, I can't. I just think it's my *duty* [my italics]. I'm a Lancashire lass; all Lancashire people are like that.'

Later on in the interview she added:

'I wouldn't let him go to St Augustine's [the local mental hospital]. I thought his place was at home. I thought as long as I had health and strength I would look after him.'

'Why?'

'I don't know . . . if I let him go I couldn't go out and enjoy myself.'

In other words, Mrs Fisher was suggesting that she was partially motivated by a sense of duty, and that if she transgressed that sense in herself, by failing to care for her husband properly or, worse still, by having him permanently removed from her care, then she would suffer from insupportable guilt feelings. By referring to her origins as a 'Lancashire lass,' Mrs Fisher was, I think, trying to claim that her sense of duty was instinctive and that its source was wholly mysterious to her. In effect she was indicating the power of ideology. Within a social-science frame of reference it would be more appropriate to describe Mrs

Fisher's sense of duty as deriving from a set of normative obligations which themselves derived from a set of socialized gender-related norms. Hence her inability to describe the origins of her strong desire to care for her husband and her reference to her potential feelings of guilt if he were ever to enter permanent residential care.

Among these four women who were most similar to the men carers, in that they too were caring for their spouses, there were, as has been mentioned, the two practising Catholics who appeared in the sample. Given their religious belief it is not surprising that both these women also described much of their motivation in terms of duty – which, as we shall see, many of the women carers did. It was also striking that these two women were the two who more or less explicitly denied that they loved their husbands and indicated that their sense of duty was their *sole* motivation. In this way they differed considerably from three of the male carers and the other two women carers who were caring for their husbands. Both these wives' husbands were suffering from severe senile dementia, and this in itself made their current relationship with their husbands extremely difficult. But they both also made it clear that, even when their husbands had been well, they considered themselves unhappily married. One of them said that her husband had always 'made my life hell', while the other spoke of her husband as 'a very difficult man'. Thus these two women, like some others in the sample, indicated how a sense of duty, derived from ideologies of whatever source, could be even stronger than other powerful emotions that might otherwise prevent them from becoming carers.

For both these women, the idea that drove them on was the dread of the guilt they thought they would feel after their husbands' death if they did not do everything within their power for their husbands. This was an idea common to many of the other women carers, some of whom, as we shall see, referred explicitly to a fear of the formal inquest and the possible public revelation that they had not done as much as they could and should. But religious belief seemed to bring with it an additional overlay of duty and a consequent fear of guilt. One of these Catholic carers (Mrs Ingram) also used her religion to interpret the process of caring in particularly interesting ways. She told me that her priest had said that this experience towards the end of her life was her 'purgatory'. When I asked her how she felt about caring for her husband, she said:

'Suggest some descriptive words! It does seem a terrific waste of my life. All relevance of time and place goes in these circumstances. It may be very very good for me – I don't know – but I do come near to failure. For one thing there are these very very long periods of silence. I'm keeping "monastic silence", without the benefit of a community. I can't even get to Mass, it's too much of a risk.'

When asked what it was that made her help her husband in the way that she did, she replied:

'Well, by temperament I'm a very faithful person. Of course I *am* a Catholic – so in any case the easier options aren't open to me. I couldn't at any stage have left him. But you're not expected by the church to hold out unreasonably. If I survive it I shall get a certain peace of mind. I won't have any feeling of guilt at all, but I shall have lost a great deal as well.'

At the end of the interview, Mrs Ingram showed me a Latin tag she had written at the front of her diary indicating that she should continue to do God's will.

Thus among the eight carers who were caring for their spouses, four of whom were men and four women, there already seemed to be major sex differences in their own descriptions of their motivation to care. While three out of the four men claimed they cared for their wives because they cared *about* them, only two of the caring wives claimed this as their motivation, and one of these indicated a mix of motives that included a strong sense of duty and potential guilt. The other two wives seemed, in contrast, to feel little love for their husbands *per se* (although see page 114 for a description of how Mrs Mitchell now loved her husband as 'another baby') but kept going because of their strong religious belief and the sense of duty derived from it.

It is, I think, significant that the word 'duty' never crossed the lips of any of the men. Even the male carer who was hoping to bring his relationship with his wife to an end by getting her permanently admitted to the local mental hospital did not mention a feeling of guilt that might ensue as a result. Instead he said that he would miss 'the company' and that he would be very lonely once he was on his own. It is almost as if the word 'duty' was missing from the men carers' vocabulary, and the sense of normative obligations, when it comes to caring, was missing from their experience. It seems, too, that the only language the men could find to explain their long-term caring behaviour was language derived from ideas of love. If this is the case, it is an important basis for the explanation of sex differences in the formation of caring relationships; for the sense of duty is generalizable from one relationship to another and it is largely unconditional; in contrast, the sense of love is highly specific to particular relationships and there is a strong element of conditionality.

Such a distinction between love and duty is not simply a researcher's artificial construct. Nor does it only arise out of the apparent gender-related differences in language and motivation of the carers looking after their spouses. Many of the women who were caring for someone other than their own spouses also clearly distinguished in their own minds between love and duty, and were often able to articulate exactly which feeling was the basis of their own motivation. There was one carer in particular (Mrs Archer) who, because she was caring for both her parents and felt very differently about each of them, was able to make clear distinctions between the calls of love and duty throughout the interview. In general Mrs Archer felt that there were certain obligations that arose regardless of the kin relationship; as a result, she greeted me at the door with the words, 'I'm a *daughter*, not a carer!' Later she said:

'To me you look after your mum and dad. A "carer" seems to be anybody. I couldn't do this sort of thing for anybody. To me it's the family. I'm a *daughter*. It's family, isn't it?'

However, at the same time, Mrs Archer made clear distinctions between the loving basis on which she cared for her mother and the dutiful basis on which she cared for her father. When asked why she helped her parents in the way that she did, she said.

'Because I love them – well, I don't always love my dad at times, but I love my mum. We have him for lunch every Sunday; that gets to be a bit of a duty. It isn't really conscience, it's because I love my mum. If anything happens to Mum I don't think I'll go and see him anything like as much.'

Thus Mrs Archer articulated the contrast between love and duty; but, unlike the two Catholic carers discussed above, she expected that, when it came to the test, her sense of duty would be less powerful than her feelings of love in terms of the services she was prepared to offer.

One other woman carer, also caring for two people, echoed Mrs Archer's views and was also able to make this kind of distinction between her feelings of duty arising out of a close family relationship and her feelings of love for someone rather more distant in terms of kin. This was Mrs Cook, who, having cared for her mother until she had died, now cared for her father and her aunt (her mother's sister). Mrs Cook cared for her father, as she put it, 'automatically', for her aunt because she loved her:

'With Dad it just sort of comes automatically. With Auntie I've just been so close to her.'

These automatic feelings as far as her father was concerned had been partially generated by her mother, who, just before she died, had said (according to Mrs Cook), 'You will take care of Father, won't you?' Mrs Cook said to me; 'And being an *only* daughter, one just automatically does.' When I asked her what satisfaction she got from the caring she did, she continued her theme of contrast between love and duty:

'Oh, it's what they give back to you! I *loved* helping my mother; that big thanks in their eyes. Father could be a bit more grateful, especially to his son-in-law.'

In contrast to Mrs Archer who did not expect her feelings of duty about her father to generate the quality of care she was prepared to offer her much loved mother, there seemed to be no discernible difference between the services which Mrs Cook was prepared to offer her father and her aunt.

Other women carers found and stated that a sense of duty based on normative obligations arising out of the family relationship was, as the Catholic women discussed above had found, enough to generate totally adequate care for their cared for. Thus Miss Nicholson, who along with her unmarried sister provided constant high-quality care for her mother, said:

'It's something to do with being a member of a family really! I don't think there's strong emotional ties; it seemed the obvious thing to do. Also, I'm very much against living on the state. I think one has a responsibility to one's family.'

Similarly, Miss Nicholson's sister had, according to Miss Nicholson, made the decision to travel over two hundred miles a week and stay with Miss Nicholson and their mother for three days a week, because 'my sister thought it a family commitment'. The bond between the elderly mother and her two independent and unmarried daughters seemed, in this case, to be based more on a willing and highly committed acceptance of an ideology of what family relationships should be like rather than on any particularly strong emotions (see page 121).

So many of the women respondents referred to 'duty' as their prime or only motivation that it would be rather long-winded to rehearse them at length here. For example, in answer to the question as to why they were caring for someone in the way that they did, Mrs Jackson (caring for her mother-in-law) said, 'I have an in-built sense of duty and responsibility.' Mrs Knowles (caring for her mother) said, 'First of all – *duty*. I'd hate her to go into a home, she'd be so unhappy. Last year she went to the Mount [an old people's home] for a month and she *hated* it. She came home completely changed.' Later on Mrs Knowles said, 'One just does look after one's parents.' Similarly, Mrs Davies, who was caring for her father-in-law, said, 'I suppose I've got a conscience. And it's the way I was brought up – you have a duty to help your relatives.'

Thus, like many of the women respondents already discussed, Mrs Jackson and Mrs Knowles also thought that the origins of their sense of duty were in some way instinctive or at least unavoidable. As I have suggested, these carers who found the origins of their sense of duty mysterious were, in effect, indicating the power of ideology. But there were other women respondents who, while referring to their sense of duty, were also well aware of where that sense came from. In particular there were three respondents who felt that the pressure to care for their parents or parents-in-law came from the cared for themselves. For example, Mrs Lee was caring for her mother who lived round the corner, and referred to her sense of duty by saying that she thought that she and her husband took their family responsibilities 'more seriously than others' and that 'all the time they're alive we should do as much as possible'. But throughout the interview Mrs Lee also indicated that her mother put very considerable pressure on her to fulfil the caring role that she expected of her.

'Mother expects it. I feel guilty if I don't go down. . . . Now I've been away so much and developed independence and I don't want to tell my mother everything. But Mother is bored. She puts the pressure on. Even when others visit she rings me up to ask why I haven't been to see her.'

When I asked her what satisfaction she got from caring, she said:

'That we're just helping. I like to think that our children would do the same for us, though I hope I'd never get as possessive as my mother! Mother punishes me for not coming every day by not speaking. The doctor says she's got coronary depression.'

Mrs Lee felt that in certain respects her mother was exerting moral blackmail. This was also the case with Mrs Green and Mrs Evans. When I asked Mrs Green what was wrong with her mother-in-law, she said emphatically, *'Nothing!'* Then, when I asked her (trying to establish whether her mother-in-law was at all confused) whether her mother-in-law knew where she was, Mrs Green said, 'She knows where she is and she knows where she's well off!' Mrs Green said her mother-in-law blackmailed her by pretending to faint and that a suitable summary of her household relations since the recent arrival of her mother-in-law was to say that 'she tyrannizes me but not my husband'. One of Mrs Green's complaints was that, despite her certainty that there was nothing wrong with her mother-in-law, the old lady did not lift a finger in the house, 'not even to peel the sprouts or clean the silver'. And Mrs Green had an interesting speculative reason as to why her mother-in-law had suddenly become so overweeningly demanding:

'She just wants me to be here and looking after her only. Whether it was because she looked after Father all those years . . .'

In other words, it may well have been the case that Mrs Green's mother-in-law was apparently being so demanding because people had expected her to provide services all her life, and she felt that now it was time for some other woman to take on these onerous tasks.

Mrs Evans, who had lived with her mother for twenty-six years, was under similar pressure; but in her case she was certain that it was because she was a woman that her mother was able to exert the pressure she did. Describing her mother as 'the matriarch round here', Mrs Evans said:

'It's become a battle of wills. She considers that daughters *should* be responsible for parents. It's not quite like that any more! She says she won't eat if she goes into Connors House [the local day centre with a few respite beds]. She'd make up her mind to die; I'd get to feel like the executioner! So I think I tend to chicken out – and, anyway, "there, but for the Grace of God . . ." '

Later she said.

'I don't feel bitter about it as such, but I do feel that we were brought up when daughters, especially the eldest daughter, were expected to look after Mother. But it's different now, though; I don't want my children to do it for me!'

It may not have been a coincidence that all three carers who described the person they were caring for as exerting considerable, and in their opinion manipulative, pressure on them were caring for women. During the interview with Mrs Evans it emerged that her mother had herself been a carer and had looked after Mrs Evans's father for long periods of his life. Thus, as with Mrs Green's mother-in-law, it is possible that here was another example of a woman carer determined, at the end of her own life, to operate a kind of surrogate and unilateral reciprocity by extracting as many caring services as possible from another younger woman in her immediate family network. But whatever the reason, there is no doubt that these three carers' sense of duty arose only partially out of a generalized idea of family obligations; of greater importance was the nature of the particular caring relationship they were engaged in and the way the person they were caring for was able to use gender-related normative obligations to generate the services they needed.

Before leaving this complicated area of the contrasts between love and duty as the prime motivators to care, it is important to stress the point that, despite the emphasis of the discussion so far, these two sets of feelings are not necessarily direct alternatives, nor static and steady states. Not only is it possible to care for someone because one feels *both* love and duty; it is also possible that out of duty grows love and that love itself can change to duty. In this sample there were two women carers who seemed to me to indicate how, at certain points in a caring relationship, the motivation to care can radically change. These were Mrs Barnes (caring for her mother-in-law) and Mrs Hall (caring for her mother). In both these cases the old ladies they were caring for were suffering from senile dementia; as a result, both their personalities had largely changed. The changes in the feelings of Mrs Barnes and Mrs Hall seemed to bear some considerable relation to the changes that had taken place in the person they were caring for. In the case of Mrs Barnes she had started to care for her mother-in-law because she had felt there was no alternative and because such care bore a close similarity to the tasks of the nursing career she had abandoned when she married (see Chapter 4 for a discussion of Mrs Barnes's construction of caring as paid work). Mrs Barnes said, at the beginning of the interview, that she looked on her caring 'as just another job'; she also had strong professionally based objections to the care her mother-in-law had received when she had spent a brief period in the local mental hospital for assessment. As Mrs Barnes herself said, 'I do take it quite seriously.' In other words, Mrs Barnes's prime motivation when she had started to care for her mother-in-law was normative obligations that derived partially from her position as daughter-in-law, but more importantly from her *dedicated professionalism*. As she put it, 'You just don't want to throw in the towel!' But something else had happened to Mrs Barnes. As her mother-in-law had grown more confused and hence dependent, Mrs Barnes had come to love her.

'I suppose I'm much closer to her than I used to be. She was very self-contained and didn't really need a daughter-in-law or friend.'

When I asked her why she helped her mother-in-law in the way she did, she said immediately:

'Oh, for someone who's so floundering. She *melts* me; she really does. It's love for her, I suppose.'

Thus, when it came to the nub of their current relationship, professionalism flew out of the window, and love flew in. Because Mrs Barnes was in any case professionally responsive to dependency, she had come to love her mother-in-law; in other words, *as a result* of caring *for* her mother-in-law, Mrs Barnes had come to care very much *about* her.

In the case of Mrs Hall, almost the reverse had been the case. Mrs Hall was one of five daughters. When it first became evident that their mother could no longer live on her own due to the onset of senile dementia, Mrs Hall had offered to have her mother live in the Halls' house. This was on the grounds that she and her mother had enjoyed a special relationship, unlike her sisters. Thus, in answer to the question as to why she helped her mother in the way that she did, Mrs Hall said:

'I don't like the thought of her being in a home. And because we've been so close. I was the favourite.'

However, due to the development of her mother's disruptive illness, Mrs Hall's relationship with her mother had drastically altered.

'I turn myself off. I can't cuddle her and kiss her like I used to. I say it's my mum's body but not my mother that's inside of it any more. Everything's the opposite to what it used to be.'

When I asked Mrs Hall why, despite her changed feelings towards her, she resisted having her mother taken permanently into residential care, she said:

'It's a decision [i.e. to no longer care informally for someone] you don't feel you can take yourself. I was made to feel extremely guilty right from the beginning. The doctor at the hospital said, "So you want to put your old mother in a home, do you?" My sisters say she should be in a home. At the moment I'd rather things carried on as they were than feel even guiltier.'

Thus, for Mrs Hall a great source of sadness was not only the change in her mother but also the change in her own feelings towards her. Love was an emotion she had given and received in the past; her present motivation was based on a sense of duty largely deriving from her perception of what others in authority might think of her should she allow her mother to be 'put away'.

To summarize this discussion of the reasons the carers themselves gave for their motivation to care and how these reasons seemed to bear some relation to the sex of the carer: I have suggested that on the whole the men carers used the language of love, while on the whole the women used the language of duty, even some of those women who were caring for their husbands. Thus the men explained their behaviour in terms of their feelings and, in particular, how they felt about the person they were caring for. In contrast, the women described their motivation in terms of obligations; those obligations were based less on the feelings that they had about the person they were caring for, and a great deal more on the obligation they felt towards their own or their husbands' kin. I suggested that these sex differences in the use of language were very significant because they meant that men's propensity to care was constrained by a more bounded set of conditions than that of women. Men would be unlikely to care for someone whom they could not legitimately claim to love on an intimate basis, while women would only be unlikely to care for someone who they felt could not make legitimate claims on their time based on kinship. Among the women carers in this sample the most prevalent claims accepted as legitimate seemed to be those of parents or parents-in-law (see Chapter 3).

A PERMANENT SOLUTION?

As should be clear by now, most of these carers had considered and rejected the possibility of permanent residential care for the person they were caring for. For almost all the men, and for the four women carers looking after their husbands, it was obvious that to place their spouse in residential care would effectively bring their marriages to an end; and they had strong opinions, based on love through to religious sanction, that they neither wanted to, nor felt they should, separate from their spouses. Thus to use the residential solution for the situation of these married carers would be to destroy what most of them considered to be their prime and lifelong committed relationship. For the carers – all of them women – who were caring for someone, usually a parent or a parent-in-law, of a different generation, other considerations prevailed. All of them felt a sense of obligation towards dependent members of their family. How they expressed that sense of obligation ranged from the reasoned argument of Miss Nicholson in support of the principle of family as opposed to state care (see pages 93–4) to the exasperated outburst of Mrs Green, who summed up the feelings of many of these women carers when she said:

'You'd feel so blasted guilty if we put her away and she died!'

Although most of these carers did, like Mrs Green, use the language of guilt to explain their motivation, particularly to carry on caring, it was nevertheless also clear that a number of them had considered the alternative of residential care very seriously. There were three main further grounds for rejecting permanent care. The first, and probably the most important, was a horror of permanent residential institutions based either on hearsay or on direct experience. For example, Mrs Evans referred to the workhouse:

'I remember my aunt dying in the workhouse. I'd rather kill myself than die in a place like that.'

Personal memories of the workhouse have become part of the British folk memory and it is possible that others among the older carers also felt a strong horror of any kind of publicly funded permanent care. However, some of the other carers had had direct and much more recent experience of residential care. Mrs Barnes reported on her mother-in-law's stay in the local mental hospital for assessment.

'My mother-in-law is now there for assessment. She's stopped speaking, she hasn't got her teeth in, and her hair hasn't been done. She's miserable there, and there's an awful stigma to mental hospitals.'

Other carers referred to the decline in the health of their cared for on their return from respite care in a local residential home, most frequently finding that their dependant was now at least disoriented and at most seriously confused. Thus one of the most important reasons for rejecting residential care, apart from guilt, was a common feeling that the quality of care the carers could themselves provide in their homes was itself considerably better than anything that could be provided by the state either in hospital or in Part III accommodation. Similar views were expressed about the relative quality of care in the private sector (a boom industry in the one-time holiday towns of East Kent). For example, Mrs Jackson, when talking about all forms of residential care, said:

'I just thought it was quite monstrous that she should go into Part III. It would have had to be somewhere in London, and we couldn't really have visited her easily. We did look at some private places round here but we didn't like them enough, really. He was happy to have her if I felt I could manage it.'

A second reason for rejecting residential care was the fear that the managers of a residential home, whether in the private or the public sector, would actually reject *them*. For example, both Mrs Davies and Mrs Barnes thought the behaviour of their parents-in-law too disruptive to be acceptable in a public institution and that therefore care in Mrs Davies's and Mrs Barnes's private homes was the only solution. Ironically, it is precisely at the point when the behaviour of their elderly dependant becomes too disruptive of family life that many carers think they might consider residential care; by then, if Mrs Davies's and Mrs Barnes's views are an accurate reflection of the reality of access to residential care, it might be too late. The final reason that one or two carers mentioned with reference to residential care was the expense of it. At present, given the provision of DHSS cover of the full costs of residential care for supplementary benefit claimants, there is a curiously polarized situation; only the very poor and the very rich can make a decision about residential care based on considerations other than the impact of the sheer expense of such care.

Given the difficulties of using residential care, it is not surprising that some of the respondents were very upset about their own feelings of revulsion towards it and, if they did not feel repelled, then about their difficulties in finding out about what was available and whether or not their cared for would be acceptable. For example, Mrs Davies spent some time during the interview worrying away at this problem.

'No ordinary residential home will have him because of his sexual problems. I won't have him in our house! Am I wrong? ... I'm very concerned about the future and getting on to waiting-lists and things. It's all so unpredictable. I do like to be prepared. Where do we go from here?'

And Mrs Evans, who had a horror of death in the workhouse, had a personal vision based on her desperation.

'My husband always says, "You'll get your thanks in heaven!" I only hope I live to see the day when the government solves this awful problem. I'd like the doctor to come in one day and say to me, "It's no longer your worry and your responsibility. We've got an answer!" But I don't think that's going to happen. And then my husband says, "What's going to happen when *you* get ill? *I* can't cope with Mother and my job!"'

6
The process of caring

Much of the interview with the carers was devoted to the process of caring: what they actually had to do in terms of housework and personal care, how they felt about doing those things, and how they felt about the person they cared for, both now and in the past. From an early stage in each interview it was usually evident that the carer had something he or she specifically wanted to tell me, or a pressing issue that they wanted to mull over with me. Thus each of the interviews tended to take on a life of its own, with the interviewee in, I hope, as strong a position as myself to decide what issues should be discussed at length.

In the following chapter I have tried to reflect these different interests and perspectives on caring but have set them within an interpretation that usually refers to how the carers seem themselves to have constructed a model and rationale of their particular caring relationship. In the case of the men, this interpretative task was relatively easy, since two of them, in particular, used the language of their previous occupations to describe the caring they did, and a third set the interview within an occupational context. For the women, interpretation was more difficult, because so many of them were prepared to talk about their feelings about caring. I was often aware that they were telling me things that had a certain historical meaning and psychological power for themselves which I could only guess at. Some of that guess-work is contained within the following pages, but during this writing-up process I have frequently felt simultaneously arrogant (to assume that I understand what these respondents were saying to me) and at a loss to understand the inner meaning of what I heard. Inevitably, the evidence and the interpretations based upon it are highly selected by myself. As with the evidence presented in Chapter 3, they should be regarded not so much as the cut-and-dried outcome of highly directed and easily managed research, but rather as tools and hypotheses on which further research can be based.

TALKING ABOUT CARING

One of the most important ways in which the men and women differed in their discussion of caring was in how they did or did not use their previous occupational experience to discuss their caring methods, in how they thought about caring, and in how they described it to me. It is perhaps inevitable, given class and sexual divisions, that of the nineteen respondents two of the men but none of the women had had professional careers: one as a top manager in a large multinational company and another as an academic and scientific attaché in the British diplomatic service. A number of the women had had careers in the para-medical professions: two as nurses, one as a pharmacist, one as a radiographer, and one as a medical secretary. Occasionally, these women carers also used their occupational experience to describe what they did, but with nothing like the intensity or consistency of the men carers.

THE MEN CARERS

Of the four men carers, one had been an academic and a scientific attaché in the Foreign Office, and another a manager in a very large multinational firm. The third had been a foreman carpenter and joiner. Only Mr Unwin had been in semi-skilled work all his life, starting off as a miner and finishing up as a doughmaker in the local bakery. The social context of the interviews themselves betrayed something of the different realms in which the men and women carers were accustomed to operate.

For example, Mr Young (the retired carpenter) sat throughout our first meeting with pencil and paper poised as if to make notes on what was said. Similarly, at our second meeting Mr Williams (the retired academic and diplomat) had made notes of the points he wished to raise at the interview and then dictated them to me. Mr Vaughan spent so long in the first interview telling me about his working life that we had hardly tackled the questions about caring when it was time for him to get ready for his wife's return from the day centre. The interviews with the one-time professional men were, out of the whole sample, the longest; they had a great deal to say about the nature of their wives' dependency and about the way they carried out their wives' care. In contrast, many of the interviews with the women carers were much more like social calls than processes whereby information was exchanged. Some of the women carers had clearly been to some trouble to provide a companionate atmosphere for the interview, underwritten by the provision of coffee and biscuits. While the interviews with all the carers were long, those with the women carers tended to be shorter than those with the men – largely, I felt, because the women carers assumed that, since I was a woman, there was little need to explain in great detail the actual process of caring.

However, even more striking than the contrast in the interview situation between business-like men and sociable women was the way similar contrasts emerged when the men and women carers came to talk about how they carried out their caring. For two of the men carers in particular, it was their work experience as, respectively, a business manager and a scientific practitioner and teacher that most seemed to inform how they carried out their caring and also how they spoke about it to me and, apparently, to others. Mr Vaughan, the retired chief accountant, was a striking example of someone who had translated concepts such as efficiency and productivity from the business world into the domestic domain. For example, before moving to Canterbury he had checked out the availability of social-service help, and once he had made the final decision to move there he had written to the local Social Services Department warning the department of their imminent arrival and of the rather frail state of his own and his wife's health. On their arrival in their new flat, Mr Vaughan had set about rationalizing the housework:

'We've tried to be intelligent about it and eliminate inessentials. We've got rid of all our brass ornaments. The other house looked as though a woman lived in it – lots of fussy little bits! I've tried to plan this flat to make it as labour saving as possible, so we've got a washing-machine and a dishwasher.'

Later he said, 'Women are naturally dextrous and better at knitting and sewing. But in principle housework isn't degrading for men; it's just a question of *efficiency* [my italics].'

Mr Vaughan had a rather elaborate system for drawing up the weekly shopping-list for their home help. But perhaps the point in the caring process where he most drew on his experience of paid work was in the management of his wife's medication. Ever since his wife had first been diagnosed as having Parkinson's disease, Mr Vaughan had kept hourly charts recording the time at which she had taken her drugs and the amount, and the timing and severity of her attacks of 'shakes'. The purpose of this was to try to assess the general efficacy of whatever drug his wife was currently prescribed and to optimize the timing and amount of drug dosage. Mr Vaughan showed me the daily records of the previous year. One of his many worries was that, should anything happen to him, his wife would have to go into permanent residential care and that she would thereby lose control of her own medication. But it later became clear that Mr Vaughan was the manager of his wife's medication:

'In our case, I'm much better at it [i.e. managing drugs]. I'm much more numerate than she is. She always used to find it difficult to control it. In the end she asked me to take over. I remind her throughout the day when she needs to take them.'

Whenever Mr Vaughan talked about matters concerning personal relationships, he used language that often directly referred to his business experience. The strength of that experience came through particularly when he talked about his own personality in contrast to that of his wife:

'She's never cross or bad-tempered. I suppose I'm male and revert to bad *business* habits and get a little impatient [my italics].'

When I asked Mr Vaughan whether he hoped or expected to receive anything in return for the caring he was doing, he once again replied in terms of the labour market:

'I don't expect to receive anything in return. It becomes something totally different if you expect a reward. Giving is giving, and *commerce* is something totally different [my italics].'

The management of his wife's illness had become his full-time retirement occupation:

'She certainly provides me with a reason for living. After so many years of retirement I'd be feeling rather useless by now. If she dies before me I now know so much about caring I'd want to carry on caring for somebody else.'

Thus Mr Vaughan had apparently translated his own personal work experience as an accountant very directly into the process of caring for his wife. This aspect of the work of caring seemed to give him some satisfaction; and he could draw comfort from the thought that through control of her medication he still apparently retained some control over the course of his wife's illness. Both household management and the management of caring in the Vaughan home bore strong parallels with his ideas of business efficiency.

The second male carer who made parallels between his own work experience and the process of caring was Mr Williams. His wife's unusual illness had started when she was relatively young and had drastically affected her memory and speech, so that for the previous four years she had not spoken at all. Mr Williams had had a long career in experimental physics, mainly as a teacher but also as a scientific attaché. It was his teaching experience which he largely brought to bear in managing his wife's illness. Thus, in describing the progression of Mrs Williams's illness, he said:

'Life continued here – my wife's mental problems getting more acute. For example, she stopped reading. She used to forget how to cook from week to week, so I used to insist on her reading recipes. I tried to keep her up to things. I wanted to learn to paint so I joined a painting class. I took her along with me, but she didn't wade in; she would just sit there eating sweets. So then I just left her at home.'

He talked about how he devised ways of keeping his wife occupied:

'I used to take her out everywhere with me. I wasn't embarrassed at all by my wife's illness. I suppose some people say she was silly, but I continued to take her everywhere with me. I took her to the theatre and the cinema at the university till the end of last term. I used to borrow big picture books for her to read, but then she used to kiss the pictures so I had to stop that. So then I used the mail-order catalogues. I found these were excellent. I just dumped them in front of her and was able to go to my Russian class.'

In some ways he regretted his somewhat schoolmasterly attitude. When I asked him whether the care of his wife presented him with any particular difficulties, he said:

'I would say this: my characteristic is that I get very impatient with people who don't do their best. I tended to get rather angry when I thought she wasn't doing her best. I used to blow up at her with her incontinence, particularly when she'd not gone to the toilet "with proper seriousness". She wouldn't even get through breakfast without being wet. I felt that really she was just not taking any trouble.'

Thus Mr Williams had adapted his lifelong experience of teaching into a mode of managing his wife's illness. His intention was to maintain his wife's skills and capacities for as long as possible by keeping them in use, and if that was against her will, then so be it.

Mr Williams was also a very active member of the Carers' Support Group. This commitment to the group was congruent with and further encouraged Mr Williams's view of himself as similar to a professional carer. The professional language of doctor and patient permeated Mr Williams's sense of his public self and that of other carers. During the interview he listed a number of points he wanted me to take note of:

'Second point: a carer must be in charge. I see some of my *colleagues* there – they're completely under the thumb of their *invalid patient.*'

And again:

'Another bee: I think you must keep the *patient* doing the absolute maximum and for as long as possible. When she broke her wrist she did nothing for about a month; she forgot practically everything then. The only things I could keep going was a bit of dusting and wiping up. She'd previously gone round with a vacuum-cleaner. About two months ago she just put the duster on her head. But she continued wiping up a bit longer but one fine day she just walked out on it [all my italics].'

Mr Williams found this professional medical language useful in explaining himself and his wife to observing strangers:

'She started doing silly things in the shops. She used to shout in the shops, "Don't hit me!" Fifteen pairs of eyes looking at the wife-beater! My wife might decide not to get on the bus and I would have to manhandle her on to it. She would follow people in the street – presumably they looked more like me than I did myself! I used to reply, "*I am a doctor and this is my mental patient*" [my italics].'

While it is perfectly understandable that Mr Williams should use this kind of language to explain himself and his wife in public, it is also important that the adoption of this language and perception of self is based on assumptions of class and gender. In other words, it would be difficult, if not impossible, for either a working-class man or most women of any class to make plausible claims to doctor status. Indeed, it is unlikely that a woman would feel the need to present any kind of explanation of her publicly observed caring behaviour.

The interviews with Mr Williams took place within a week or so of Mrs Williams's death. Mr Williams was already beginning to think tentatively about how he might spend his time in future. It was not surprising to learn that he hoped to get involved with the after-care of stroke patients at the local hospital and that he intended to continue to go to the Carers' Support Group. Mr Williams, like Mr Vaughan, had found by force of circumstance that caring had had to become his full-time retirement occupation. But out of their personal difficulties Mr Williams and Mr Vaughan were well aware that they had acquired interests, experience, and knowledge that they felt could be usefully extended to help others in similar situations to themselves and their wives. Once again, there may well be underlying issues of gender here; for I think it unlikely that many women would be so aware that they had, through the process of caring, acquired a body of knowledge that was transmittable and transferable to other carers. The only comparable woman in this particular sample was Mrs Barnes, whom I have elsewhere described as a 'career' carer (see Chapter 4). It was her original occupational training as a nurse that made her sensitive to the fact that the experience of caring constitutes a set of skills and creates a body of knowledge. In the same way, these two men, as a result of having had to learn these skills 'from scratch' as it were, were also aware that they had become 'retirement' carers. Their use of language, derived from the labour market and from professional occupations, combined with the use of their personal work experience to inform their own methods of caring, indicated that they perceived caring as similar to paid and, to some extent, prestigious labour.

The other two men in the sample – Mr Young and Mr Unwin – were retired from skilled and semi-skilled manual occupations and hence not on the whole able to use the largely class-based models of professional care that were accessible to Mr Vaughan and Mr Williams. Nevertheless Mr Young also described his wife as a patient, saying, 'Most of the time she's a very good patient but sometimes she rebels.' Mr Young was also very concerned about the management of his wife's medication and felt strongly that this was his special sphere of care for his wife. However, Mr Unwin, in contrast to the other three men, who all took a very positive view of their personal competence to care, seemed to be rather upset. Part of Mr Unwin's problem was that, in marked contrast to the other men carers, he was getting no Social Services help whatever. It was not as though he could manage on his own. He found it very difficult to bath his wife by himself, particularly as she often refused to co-operate. He found her incontinence and loss of ability to eat with utensils distressing and disgusting; with no washing-machine, he had to wash all their bed linen and clothes by hand. The control of his wife's medication, rather than being welcome and a self-conferred source of status, caused him considerable anxiety; he was very worried the day I saw him that, with a new prescription, he had given his wife an overdose of a sleeping-draught. Throughout the interview he referred to the fact that he often got 'nasty' with his wife and that this too worried him a great deal. It is not therefore surprising that Mr Unwin was hoping to get his wife into permanent residential care at the earliest possible moment. Of all the carers interviewed in this sample, Mr Unwin was the most desperate and the one for whom the Social Services provided the least. He was a man at sea, forced to do something at which he felt totally incompetent and from which he could derive no satisfaction.

THE WOMEN CARERS

The contrast between the men and women carers when it came to talking about the caring they did was striking. As was pointed out above, three of the men were eager to discuss the techniques of caring in order to demonstrate their newly acquired skills. The women carers, on the other hand, were less inclined to talk about the techniques of caring – possibly because they thought there was 'nothing' to them, especially when being interviewed by another woman. However, the women were on the whole rather more voluble than the men about the particular difficulties of caring and the emotional problems their caring had caused, or in one or two cases, was designed to resolve.

Before carrying out the interviews, I had hypothesized that the women carers would refer to their actual or potential experience as mothers to describe the caring they did (Ungerson 1983b). In the questionnaire I included questions and possible prompts asking all the respondents whether they felt 'maternal' about the person they were caring for. Some of them said they did, but far more said they did not. While there were women who had evidently constructed their caring relationship as a maternal one, there were others for whom the maternal model was not only inappropriate but also made them feel distinctly uncomfortable. Far more striking, when looking at the contrast between the men and women carers, was the relative homogeneity of the men's language and its occupational reference, compared to the heterogeneity of the women's language and perception. The one thing the women had in common was their rather more general willingness – and need – to talk about their feelings about caring.

In the following section an attempt will be made to tease out some of these emotional aspects and consequences of caring by looking at women caring for people in a particular kin or marital relation to themselves: their husbands, their own mothers or fathers, and their parents-in-law. However, during this discussion it should also become clear that, while there are important issues arising out of the particular kin relationship of woman carer and cared for (particularly the question of power between daughters and mothers and daughters-in-law and their mothers-in-law), an equally important determinant of how the women carers felt about their caring was probably whether or not they had other people, such as husbands and children, also dependent on their wifely and mothering services.

Women caring for their husbands

In this sample there were four women caring for their husbands. The youngest was in her late fifties, the oldest in her mid-seventies. Two of them (Mrs Ingram and Mrs Mitchell) were caring for one-time professional men who had recently become very seriously ill with senile dementia. The other two (Mrs Fisher and Mrs Osborne) were caring for husbands who had been seriously disabled nearly all or, in the case of Mrs Osborne, all their married lives. Thus Mrs Ingram and Mrs Mitchell had each recently experienced very considerable change in the nature of their relationship with their husbands, while both Mrs Fisher and Mrs Osborne had been their husbands' carers for many decades. In the case of Mrs Fisher, whose husband had had a cerebral haemorrhage early in their marriage, the need for adjustment to changed circumstances had long since passed. As Mrs Fisher put it when I asked her whether she had any difficulties about caring, 'I've done it for so long now I just take it in my stride.'

The one thing that really worried Mrs Fisher was the state of health of her 90-year-old mother, who lived alone in Lancashire. If her mother were to become so ill that she needed full-time care, Mrs Fisher dreaded the possibility that, in order to care for her mother, she might have to arrange for her husband to go into the local mental hospital in the interim, and once there 'the hospital might not let him out'. She was also very worried that she might never see her mother again. In the two weeks before the interview, Mr Fisher had had a number of *grand mal* fits, and Mrs Fisher chose to interpret this as a symptom of her husband worrying about his future care should she need to go to Lancashire to look after her mother. Much of the interview was taken up with Mrs Fisher talking about this problem of the competing needs of her two nearest and dearest. In this, Mrs Fisher had much in common with other women carers, discussed below, who were also very concerned about other elderly people in their immediate kin network who needed them but for whom they were unable to do anything.

Like Mrs Fisher, Mrs Osborne also took a very stoical attitude to her husband's disability and the caring work she had to do. In this case, her husband, who was present at the interview, seemed to be more concerned than she was that he go into respite care in order for her to have a holiday and a complete rest from caring. It seemed to me that for these two women, each of whose lives had been deeply affected by their husband's disability but who had also had decades to become accustomed to it, their stoicism had combined with immutable circumstances to make apparently very successful caring relationships.

In contrast, for Mrs Ingram and Mrs Mitchell the problem was not how to make sense of lack of change, but rather how to cope with fundamental and recent change. Both could be said to have suffered some of the consequences of a bereavement, and in certain respects their reaction to the loss of their husbands was somewhat similiar. As 'quasi-widows' they had both lost a partner who had, according to their own descriptions of their marriages up to the point of their husbands' illness, been dominant and even domineering. Now the boot was on the other foot, and they both had had to adjust to becoming *de facto* heads of household. Neither woman had ever been responsible for the administrative details of running a household, and one of them said that, far from having to manage the household finances, her husband had kept her very short of money: 'He wouldn't let me near his money. All I was there for was to do all the chores.' Thus one of their new problems was concerned with having to take responsibility for financial matters. For Mrs Mitchell this had proved to be a source of great satisfaction, since somewhat to her surprise she had discovered that she was rather good at household administration; she had managed to make up the full grants of her student children, complete the tax form, and make a small surplus over the previous year. Mrs Ingram, however, had found the adjustment to household head far more difficult. When I asked her what changes she had had to make to her life as a result of her husband's illness, she said:

'Of course now I have an enormous workload – things like repairing, administration, budgeting. Now if there's anything that's got to be done I've got to do it. I didn't drive or even open a car door for years!'

Later in the interview, when I asked her how she felt about being the person who gave most help to her husband, she said:

'It's completely unnatural to me. On the whole I've always received more help than given it. It's a reversal of role as far as I'm concerned. My friends have always been pretty protective on the whole; I gave the impression of being an idiotic type. I can't deal with the insurance [her cellar had been flooded when a sewer had burst]. I can't cope, and that's that. I haven't sent in a claim or anything.'

Mrs Ingram, therefore, was having some difficulties in adjusting to her new position as head of the household. She had been a protected wife, and believed explicitly in a conventional sexual division of labour:

'I think it's one of the modern heresies that everyone can do everything. I think there are sex differences and divisions. A man tends to shove housework off on to shopkeepers and restaurants and things. A woman also has a willingness which leads to experience. There has to be a division of labour because of the lack of time. No one person can do everything.'

It is interesting that, where a conventional view of the relations between married couples prevails, it seems to be more difficult in certain respects for married women to adjust to caring for their husbands than it is for married men to adjust to caring for their wives. One might expect the opposite to be true – namely, that married men who believe in a conventional sexual division of labour would find the responsibility for housework and personal care particularly difficult. However, the examples of the successful married men carers in this sample, taken with the example of Mrs Ingram, seem to indicate that there is a conventional model of the marriage relationship which makes it easier for married men to adjust to change in the circumstances of their marriages than it is for married women. This is the model of the husband who, familiar with the world of the public domain, is in a position to protect his wife whose chief skills and femininity lie in the private domain of hearth and home. In important ways, this protective model of marriage is appropriate when it comes to married men caring for highly dependent wives. Despite their changed circumstances, there can remain a continuity in the idea of protection, and it can even be further developed without threatening either the husband's masculinity or his wife's femininity. The wife is even more contained within the home, and the husband can, if he wants, find a new role in the public world as a negotiator of services for his wife. However, for a caring wife no such convenient model derived from the conventional view of marriage presents itself. Instead, she finds herself in a 'Catch 22' situation, where to be 'uncaring' would be to be 'unfeminine', and yet to be a *competent* carer in both the private and the public domains, and hence fully protective of her husband, would also impugn her femininity.

It is perhaps no coincidence, therefore, that of all the women carers in this sample, it was one of the women caring for her husband who had adjusted to change by adopting wholesale and with zeal the mothering model of caring. This was Mrs Mitchell, whose personal circumstances were in many respects very similar to those of Mrs Ingram. Rather than struggle, as Mrs Ingram was doing, with direct role reversal as prescribed by a model of conventional marriage, Mrs Mitchell had instead found a model based, not on the marriage relationship, but on motherhood:

'We had a very stormy marriage, but now I love looking after him. Now I've got another baby; it's the same thing, really. I take a long time over his toilette. I take great pleasure in doing all these things for him.'

During the interview this motherhood model was highly evident. While we talked, Mrs Mitchell brushed her husband's hair and cleaned and polished his fingernails. Her translation from somewhat downtrodden wife (according to what she herself told me) to a highly competent and even *pleased* carer seemed to be predicated on the new roles of mother and baby that she had found for herself and her husband. As she said more than once, 'It's like having another baby again.'

It may have been no coincidence that Mrs Mitchell had had seven children and that therefore she found the motherhood model of caring very easy to adopt and one where she felt highly competent. In contrast, when I asked Mrs Ingram whether she felt maternal about her husband, she said with some vehemence:

'Frankly, I hated looking after a baby. I felt like a goat. I found it offensive, and the nappy business was revolting – it put me off it for life!'

And then she added:

'No, I don't feel maternal about him. It's a maternal type of care, but I'm not aware of having any maternal feelings for him. . . . I don't think I've got many feelings about him. I was very, very sorry at first because I think it's a terrible thing to happen to a talented man. But now I've withdrawn; it's been gradual and essential. I'd look after anybody who was in that state if I were in the same house.'

It is possible that the adoption of the motherhood model of caring had given Mrs Mitchell the space in which she felt she could control her husband and their lives together.

'It's amazing how you adjust to each new thing. I thought I'd never cope with incontinence. Now it's amazing what I can get up to. I think he's very, very good. I have to pull him around a lot, and he doesn't mind. He does give me the odd swipe, though. You can't expect to feel sweetness and light all the time. I do now more than I did. I didn't feel disgusted by incontinence for very long – only a week or two. You have to accept that he's never going to get better. The hardest thing is accepting that.'

In contrast, Mrs Ingram felt unhappy about the lack of control over her circumstances and the routines of her new life:

'I'm really quite a good nurse, oddly enough! That part doesn't worry me, as a matter of fact. I cope with that kind of physical thing reasonably well. It's a ''proper'' thing. I don't regard it as derogatory to my dignity. But it's the pacing of it. I spend most of my life waiting for things: the district nurses; for him to come out of the bathroom. And there are so many things I can't do; I can't put screws in.'

To conclude this section: these two married women caring for their husbands demonstrated the classic truism that change can be both liberating and disorienting. But I have also argued that they demonstrated how caring can be made easier if the carer successfully reconstructs the nature of her relationship with her husband into a model with which she is comfortable and to which she is accustomed. In the context of a wife caring for her husband, this model is likely to be the motherhood model. It does not threaten her identity as female or his identity as male and it is highly appropriate to the caring work she has to do.

However, where a woman carer identifies herself solely as the new head of the household, particularly where this is incompatible with relations that prevailed within the household before the onset of her husband's illness, then caring becomes more difficult since aspects of it necessarily involve becoming 'masculine'. Of course, it will always be necessary for women carers who, as a result of their husband's mental and physical incapacities, are 'quasi-widows' to adopt, and adapt to, radical changes in running the household and in particular to enter the public domain of household administration. I am arguing, however, that important questions of self-image interpose themselves in the adjustment process and that the adoption of one particular self-image and mode of relationship (that of mothering) may make these adjustments easier since it is uniquely compatible with femininity.

Women caring for a parent

In this sample there were six women caring for their own mother and one woman caring for her own father. It was perhaps these respondents who expressed some of the strongest and the most complicated feelings about the caring that they did. It is also significant in my view that many of these carers said (echoing Mrs Ingram, discussed above) that they could care only if they cut themselves off from feeling altogether and simply got on with the immediate tasks at hand. In other words, in order to care *for* their parents they found it easier to forget about caring *about* them, since some of their emotions were too distressing.

The general reason as to why these relationships seemed to be among the more complicated, and sometimes the more stressful, is almost certainly that they were the relationships with the longest histories. All these women carers had been brought up by their own parents and, with the exception of two (Mrs Lee and Miss Nicholson), had lived with or very near their parents throughout their adult lives. As a result of these very long antecedents the nature of the relationship between carer and cared for had had inevitably to change as, first, the growing child developed into an independent adult, and then the parent later changed into that child's dependant. As I have argued elsewhere, caring relationships which have a very long biography are bound to be affected by their histories; the quality of the caring relationship will be determined not only by how carer and cared for feel about each other now but also by how they have felt about each other in the past, and by how successfully changes in that relationship have been negotiated in the past (Ungerson 1983b).

There are analogies here with long-standing marriages. The history of marriages will also have a considerable bearing on how successfully they are turned into caring relationships. However, I suggested above that where caring occurs between spouses there are certain models of the marriage relationship – the protective husband, the mothering wife – that allow caring to be compatible with continuities of marriage. There seems to be no such compatible model for child/parent caring. These relationships involve a complete reversal of dependency: from child to quasi-parent and from parent to quasi-child. The only model that seems to be available under these circumstances, especially where the carer is a daughter, is that of mothering: the biological child 'mothers' the biological parent. Just as when a wife cares for her husband, such a model is compatible with the carer's femininity. But there will be gender differences that will determine how far that motherhood model can be utilized successfully. It may be possible for a daughter carer to 'mother' her own father successfully, since the acceptance by men of the caring services of women is so commonplace (although see below for some of the problems that can arise in such a translation); but where the carer is the daughter and the cared for the mother, then there are likely to be particularly stressful problems of role reversal. It is not surprising, therefore, that either the daughters in this sample withdrew from certain aspects of caring altogether, or the successful caring daughters (and daughters-in-law) reported that they could care for their mother (or mother-in-law) only if they cut themselves off from feeling altogether and preferred to think of themselves as something more like a nurse than a close relative, let alone a mother.

Given the ages of most of these women caring for their parents, almost all of them had been in some kind of a relationship with their parent for over fifty years. That is a goodly space for all sorts of feelings – good and bad – to develop. For some of these carers, the only way they claimed that they could carry on was by ignoring their feelings or burying them. In some cases the feelings were particularly poignant, because the carer could remember how good the relationship had been before the onset of her parent's illness; in other relationships, the carer referred to long-standing difficulties with her parent which had been exacerbated by the change in their circumstances together; and in yet others, both carer and cared for apparently found it especially difficult to accept the change from parent to quasi-child and vice versa. In other words, it seems to me that when carers claimed that feelings could be obstructive rather than helpful in the caring relationship, they were also saying that they were positively hindered by the history of their relationships.

Mrs Hall, who cared for her 76-year-old mother (early senile dementia), demonstrated many of these difficulties arising out of a long history. Her relationship with her mother had been particularly close (see page 98 for an earlier discussion of how Mrs Hall came to be chief carer). When I asked her whether caring for her mother presented her with any difficulties, she said:

'Oh, it upsets me. I've turned myself off, really. I don't think she's my mum, really. We were always so close. If I wasn't well she'd come and look after the family; she used to do everything.'

Mrs Hall was very worried by this change in her relationship with her mother, particularly because her mother was now aggressive towards her. She had asked her mother's hospital consultant to explain her mother's behaviour, and he, too, had chosen to emphasize their personal biography together:

'She's very incontinent, very confused. A bit on the militant side: she flies at me. I've always been very close to her. They explained at the hospital that it's because she feels safe with me that she flies at me rather than anyone else.'

The emotional difficulties between Mrs Hall and her mother meant that she found it impossible to do any personal caring tasks for her mother. Mrs Hall's mother refused to allow her to wash her hair or bath her, and, as Mrs Hall put it:

'I've said several times that it's worse than having a baby because you can't make an adult do what you want whereas you can a child.'

Mrs Hall had managed to resolve this problem of being unable to carry out personal care by using the attendance allowance to employ a neighbour to care for her mother (see page 38). Nevertheless, the emotional difficulties were kept at bay only with great effort; she also knew that, if she visibly broke down, then the entire caring process would be put in jeopardy. When I asked her what satisfaction she got from the caring she did, she said:

'I don't get any satisfaction. If I thought about it too much I'd just sit and cry. If my husband saw me in tears, that would be the final straw.'

Thus Mrs Hall demonstrated how a close emotional relationship based on a long history together could be the initiating basis for a caring relationship – only, paradoxically, to become a source of considerable difficulty in actually carrying out personal care. The only way these difficulties could be even partially resolved was to eliminate the element of feeling (or caring *about*) from the relationship and simply get on with caring *for* the elderly person. The relationship was no longer based on historical feeling but rather on normative obligation arising out of kinship. Further obligations to other members of the family – in this case, the husband – largely forbade the expression of feelings to those who did not share, in its full intensity, the historical biography existing between mother and daughter.

Mrs Knowles also found that she had to cut herself off from feeling in order to care for her mother. Throughout the interview she stressed the difficulty that feeling could engender in any caring relationship, particularly where that feeling arose out of a long biography together. For example, towards the end of the interview I asked most of the respondents to think about some examples of kin caring for each other and to consider whether they would give rise to any particular difficulties. (These questions were really meant to get at the possible impact of incest taboos on caring, but they didn't work very well and so are not discussed in detail in this book.) When asked to consider a relationship of a daughter caring for her mother-in-law, she said:

'In a more distant relationship I think it's easier. I feel I could do more personal things for a complete stranger far easier than for a mother-in-law. I suppose I'm thinking of my relationship with my own mother-in-law. An in-law would be rather difficult;

it's not an honest relationship. One would feel even more guilty about it. . . . The difficulty is trying to let a person have their independence and dignity. With a stranger you can be more detached perhaps.'

It was possibly as a result of the difficulties that had arisen for Mrs Knowles in caring for her mother that she had come to the view that feelings and a long biography were positively obstructive to caring. Like Mrs Hall, Mrs Knowles had complicated and somewhat distressing feelings about her mother, although these had arisen out of a long history of difficulty:

'I don't think I've ever confided in her. She's always been a very negative person. She's never supported me in anything I've wanted to do.'

So for Mrs Knowles the emotional difficulties stemmed from regret not so much that she had lost, through a change of personality arising out of illness, a much loved mother, but rather that she and her mother had never had a particularly good relationship. The result, however, was the same as with Mrs Hall; Mrs Knowles found herself unable to carry out personal care tasks for her mother, particularly washing her.

'I don't wash her. I feel I could cope with somebody else's mother better than my own. I don't know why, really.'

When I asked her to consider why she felt like she did about personal caring for her mother, she said, 'We're a family who've always repressed our emotions', and later, when I asked her in more detail about the personal care she gave her mother, she referred to their biography together.

'As children I suppose we never saw our parents naked. I think my own children would be different about our nudity.'

The problem about bathing had been resolved by Mrs Knowles's woman GP arranging for her to have a district nurse visit three times a week.

Mrs Knowles and Mrs Hall were the only carers caring for someone in their own homes who had found that their feelings about the person they were caring for prevented them from carrying out essential personal tasks. Other carers referred to their need to bury their feelings in order to do the things they had to do, but they 'simply' got on with it. For example, Miss Nicholson – who, like Mrs Hall and Mrs Knowles, cared for her co-resident mother – said:

'I do think sometimes that a very strong emotional tie can interfere with caring. One's really got to be a little detached. If you link everything too closely it gets out of proportion, there's an overlay of anxiety.'

Interestingly, of all the women carers, Miss Nicholson's view of caring most nearly echoed that of the men carers described above. She tended to use the language and concepts derived from her professional life – that of a medical secretary – to say the things about caring that she felt were important, and she found intensely practical solutions for the emotional problems that arose between herself and her mother. For example, when I asked her at the end of the interview whether there was anything that she would like Social Services to do, she said:

'I think what's missing is a peripatetic physiotherapist. She'd take it better from a professional. If I tell her to stand up straight she says, "Oh, don't go on at me!"'

It seems to me ironic that precisely the elements of informal care that are supposed to be its advantages – namely, that people are cared for by those who are familiar to them and care about them – are exactly those elements that these women carers claimed were a positive hindrance to caring. In the case of Mrs Hall and Mrs Knowles these elements prevented them from the full range of caring tasks, so that Mrs Knowles had had to make considerable calls on the district nurse services and Mrs Hall had had to call on the almost constant services of an elderly neighbour. While there were particular elements to Mrs Knowles's and Mrs Hall's distress at personal care, there were also generalizable feelings of embarrassment arising out of the social mores dominant at the time when their parents were bringing them up. Other respondents also mentioned that either they or their parents found the necessity of them seeing their parents naked very embarrassing. For example, Mrs Archer said of her mother:

'Mum's a sweetie. She is embarrassed – she won't let me give her a bath, and Peter [Mrs Archer's husband] has to go out of the room. They just don't like people seeing them with no clothes on, and I get a bit embarrassed too.'

In this context some carers also said that they thought the greater laxity about nakedness that now prevailed in their immediate family would help matters if and when they themselves needed personal care from their children. Thus both personal and public elements of a long-term kin relationship could have their own inhibiting and obstructive effects on the caring process. It is ironic that it is precisely this kind of very close kin relationship that is expected by Social Service allocators to be the least problematic!

So far we have discussed the complexity of the relations between caring daughters and dependent mothers in terms of their long history together and the *continuities* of difficulty arising therefrom. But it also seemed to me that there were likely to be conflicts arising out of the *change* in their status from daughter to carer and from mother to dependant. In particular, I expected there to be problems about power. Especially where daughter and mother were living in the same household, I expected there to be power conflicts over the traditional women's domain of home and housework and that these power conflicts would also feature in the caring relationship itself. Certainly these daughters were themselves aware that there were potential and actual problems about the change in their power position *vis-à-vis* their mothers. For example, Miss Nicholson said, when considering whether there were likely to be any general difficulties about a daughter caring for her mother:

'If one character's more dominant than the other. I think really to care adequately . . . if the sick person is the dominant character, then that's very difficult. After all, you must have a pattern in caring. If you had someone who was always dictating what they wanted, life could be very unhappy.'

But Miss Nicholson's mother had hated Miss Nicholson having to take over all household tasks. When I asked Miss Nicholson how they shared the cooking and the cleaning, she said:

'One of the things that upset her so much was seeing me doing it. We now have someone to clean for her, and I do as little as possible. She worried and worried about our [Miss Nicholson and her sister were joint carers] doing her housework. She pays for the cleaner out of the attendance allowance.'

Miss Nicholson's mother, just like her daughter, also seemed to have a robustly practical answer for emotional problems! (See above, page 121.)

Among these carers looking after their mothers there were

others who found the power relationship particularly difficult to handle and not amenable to such practical solutions, largely because the person they were caring for would not go along with them. Mrs Evans, who described her mother more than once as a 'matriarch' (see page 96), was an upset and depressed carer whose mother had lived with her and her husband for twenty-six years. The relationship between Mrs Evans and her mother was an unhappy one, and Mrs Evans was very lonely:

'I'm very much on my own, and that seems to be when Mother's at her worst. . . . I suppose I'm nine-tenths on the way to being a prisoner. I can't trust her on her own any more – particularly at night. I ask a neighbour to look out for her whenever I go out. She opens the door to anyone. You're always anxious, she was lying in the garden one day when I came home. My husband gets a little disillusioned. He gets rather upset I can't go with him unless I book Connors House [the local-authority unit for respite care]. She *won't* get into a wheelchair! And that's the only way we can get out with her. . . .

'I think the worst thing I find . . . less and less contact with neighbours and people. I can cope with that provided I can paint or read, but now she doesn't like me to do that. I can go a whole week and not hold a conversation! I'm going sort of senile myself! It's made me dread getting old myself. I never see a neighbour or a member of the family – they're all over the world. You feel you're cut off from all sorts of things, especially conversation. And at night it's the loneliness and the lack of contact with people. When my husband's here, that helps. But he's away so much. He can't give up his job, so there's no choice.'

The worst problem for Mrs Evans was the guilt she felt about how her mother's presence had constrained her marriage and the power clash between herself, her mother, and her husband:

'I think he [her husband] has the worst end of the frustration, because I can't travel with him. I feel I can take much more than he can because he feels that our lives have been so restricted. I'm the bone in the middle! You're pulled both ways – he feels we haven't had a proper married life. We had our first holiday alone together two years ago, when Connors House took Mother. Previously we've always had to take Mother with us. . . .

'In fact you're still their little girl in many ways, and *he* has no right to have *his* say. There used to be arguments about it. She used to criticize but not now. She does say, "You think more of him than you do me and you were *mine* before you were *his*!" She likes to assert her authority sometimes. I think he's a brick, actually. It could have been very difficult at times if he hadn't been more easy-going.'

Asked if there were any personal care tasks with which she had particular difficulty, she said:

'Not normally, but we do get days when she'll resist anything I try and do for her, especially with personal hygiene or with her clothes.'

A little later she added, 'I think they're worse than children, because with a child you're protective but you're in *control*. But with an elderly person they fight you every inch of the way. You can't put her in a playpen or strap her into a chair.'

Thus this caring relationship was clearly a very bad one. This partly reflected the long history between mother and daughter – a fact that her mother apparently referred to, saying that her daughter was 'hers' before she was 'his' – but also reflected the relationship difficulties between the three adults that had arisen during the period of twenty-six years over which the caring had stretched. It was not surprising that Mrs Evans said towards the end of the interview:

'I'm quite certain that much as our children love us they won't do it for me. It puts a terrible strain on a marriage. I admire our kids for saying, "no, we won't do it". I think money should be spent to make sure children don't have to do it. We love our mothers – we all do – but we don't have to spend our lives paying them back!'

Other respondents also found that power relations were especially problematic. For example, Mrs Knowles told me that her mother often complained to her that 'You treat me like a child', and she was having great difficulty dissuading her mother from eating too much and drinking too much alchohol:

'I'm very concerned about the weight she's putting on. It's not good for her to have all these things. It's very difficult to say "no". She'd get through a bottle of sherry a day if she could. Sherry depresses her anyway.'

As a result of her mother's weight gain, Mrs Knowles had had to buy her a completely new wardrobe. Her mother had been unable to come to the shops with her, so Mrs Knowles had bought the dresses on her own. During the interview her mother emerged from her 'granny annexe' and could be distinctly heard outside the door of Mrs Knowles's sitting-room, shouting, 'I *hate* this dress!' Her mother also strongly objected to Mrs Knowles leaving her alone to go to a voluntary job:

'She keeps saying to me, "Are you going to that place?" and "Why don't you get a paid job?"'

Other caring daughters also reported that their mothers were very possessive of their time. For example, Mrs Lee, whose mother didn't live with them but very close by, found that her mother wanted her to be with her far more than Mrs Lee thought was necessary, and that her mother refused to use a wheelchair which might have given her some independence from Mr and Mrs Lee:

'We borrowed a wheelchair from a friend. But she *hates* it. She still thinks she can do everything and she can't. It causes friction amongst us. Dad won't take Mum out in the wheelchair, and so my husband takes them out in our car.'

Thus some carers, particularly Mrs Evans, had considerable problems around the issue of power when it came to caring for their mothers. I have no doubt that most of these difficulties had their origin in the long history of the relationship between the daughters and their mothers and in the fact that altered circumstances entailed a radically changed relationship. But it is also noteworthy that one or two daughters-in-law caring for their mothers-in-law also reported power problems (see below). It may, therefore, be possible that these difficulties also had their roots in the fact that two women were sharing a home and that it was rivalry in the domestic domain that underlay much of this trouble. This is a question which will come up again when we consider caring relations between in-laws.

In the introduction to this section, I suggested that there might be particular problems about daughters caring for their mothers which would not arise for a daughter caring for her father. This was because there would be no overt problems between a father and a daughter about power in the domestic domain and because a man would almost certainly be accustomed to, and comfortable about, receiving the services of another woman. Of these women who were caring for one of their own parents, there was only one who was caring for her father. This was Mrs Cook, who had first become a carer when she looked after her mother during her terminal illness; since her mother's death, she had become increasingly involved in caring for her mother's elderly sister and, more recently, her very elderly father. Although neither her father nor her aunt lived permanently in the Cook household, her father had recently spent six weeks recovering from pleurisy in Mrs Cook's house. At the time of the interview, the old man had returned to his own home in a nearby village, but Mrs Cook was concerned that he could not remain on his own and at such a distance from her very much longer. Mrs Cook did not seem to have any particular language or role model reference to describe the enormous amount of caring that she did. She simply got on with it, feeling that she had to and that she was good at it. She talked a lot about her motivation and the sense of duty that devolved upon women to care for their kin (see above, page 50). There was only one problem about the care that she currently did for her father – she felt that he took it for granted and did not show his gratitude enough.

At the time of the interview Mrs Cook was really doing all her father's housework and managing his rather large garden; she was doing no direct personal care. Nevertheless she had given the prospect of personal care some considerable thought. When I asked her whether her father could take himself to the lavatory, she said:

'That's the one thing that sort of worries me. This is the one thing that I'm really dreading. My husband has taken him to the loo the few times it's been necessary.'

'*Why does it embarrass you?*'

'It's because he's my *father*. It's my embarrassment for him, not so much my own embarrassment.'

'*Why is it different for father compared to mother?*'

'I don't know. I've tried to reason it out. I think he would be embarrassed.'

'*Was your mother embarrassed?*'

'At first she said it was terrible but after a while she got over it. She loved her baths. She was a very clean sort of person.'

In this way Mrs Cook echoed the words of Mrs Hall and Mrs

Knowles, neither of whom had been able to take on the most personal care for their mothers. Mrs Cook had evidently been able to resolve this as far as her own mother was concerned, but her father seemed to her to pose additional problems. Once again, my view is that these problems of personal care arise largely between kin who have a long shared biography. But in this case of a daughter caring for her father, I also think that she confirms my own hypothesis, outlined in an article written years before this study (Ungerson 1983b), that there would be additional problems of personal care where carer and cared for were close kin, related by blood, and of the opposite sex. My suggestion in that article was that there would be difficulties arising out of the operation of the incest taboos. While nothing of any generalizable significance can be made out of this single instance appearing in such an unrepresentative sample, I nevertheless present it here as possible confirmation of my original hypothesis.

It is at any rate another example of real problems of personal care between people who are biologically related and who have known each other over long periods but under very different circumstances. In some cases these difficulties may be lessened if there is (as there seems to have been in Mrs Cook's relationship with her late mother) real love and affection between carer and cared for, such that any distress over personal care can eventually evolve into something less problematic. But for others the problem could be resolved only by adopting a distancing model of care such as the occupational one of nurse (Miss Nicholson), or by engaging in open warfare (Mrs Evans), or by giving up personal care altogether (Mrs Hall and Mrs Knowles).

There is one further general point to be made about these married women caring for a parent, particularly as there are clear similarities between these daughters and the daughters-in-law considered in the next section. All these women were very concerned about the impact of their caring on the rest of their family. In other words, they were riddled with guilt. It was guilt that very largely motivated them to care and to keep on caring (see pages 90–101), but it was ironic and paradoxical that the very act of assuaging that motivating guilt created further guilt *vis-à-vis* other members of their families, notably their husbands and, where there were any, their children. As we have seen, Mrs Evans felt dreadful about the way she had deprived her husband of a 'proper married life' and that the only holiday they had ever had alone was two years previously when her mother had, for once and never again, agreed to go into respite care. Similarly, Mrs Knowles felt that her children had been deprived of a 'normal' family upbringing and that her husband was losing out on the companionate aspects of marriage. If she did go out with her husband she said she had an 'awful guilty conscience about leaving the children in charge'. Mrs Hall felt acutely sorry for her husband having to put up with her mother's incontinence and the domestic disruption that it caused. Mr and Mrs Archer, who were both present at the interview, had an argument in my presence as to how dependent Mrs Archer's parents were, with Mr Archer claiming that they did not need as much help as his wife was providing for them and that, according to Mr Archer, her 'family' needed Mrs Archer just as much. At this, Mrs Archer burst into tears. (See page 55 for a further discussion of the negotiation process involved in becoming a carer.) Mrs Cook, in order to fulfil all her domestic duties to her husband, her father, and her aunt and uncle, had the most extraordinarily attenuated day, starting off at 5 a.m. and finishing at 11.30 at night. Her own brother accused her of enjoying being a 'martyr'! Of these married women, only Mrs Lee seemed to feel no especial guilt about neglecting the rest of her family. In general, she thought that her mother's demands for visits and outings were rather too much for all the family including herself and her husband, and that her mother was successful in making them all feel guilty; she appreciated very much the help her husband gave her. Only Miss Nicholson seemed totally guilt-free. She had no husband or children to stake additional claims to her attention and services, and she had come to a formal agreement with her sister that they would share the care of their mother exactly fifty/fifty.

These 'guilty women' evidently felt that there was a prevailing hierarchy of demands which they were not fulfilling. In other words, they all thought that their own husbands and children had more legitimate claims on them than their parents did, but that the time and responsibility needed to care for an elderly person prevented them from being 'proper' wives and mothers to their more immediate nuclear family. These feelings of guilt are unlikely to besiege a male carer. All these women perceived themselves as the pivot of their immediate domestic domains, and it was their effective absence from that domain for long periods of time which made them feel guilty. It is interesting that, while policy-makers may have a view of the *extended* family as the most suitable place for the care of the elderly, it seems that married women carers of the elderly feel that such care is potentially destructive of the *nuclear* family of which they are part; care for elderly dependants prevents them from being either 'normal' mothers or 'proper' wives. These expressions of abnormality and inappropriateness tend to put into perspective the frequently made claims of politicians and social critics, particularly those on the 'new right', that family care is so normal that it must be 'natural'. What these women carers were saying was that, while it fulfilled their sense of duty to their parents, it certainly did not seem *normal* to them, and that it prevented what would otherwise have been the more natural progression of close nuclear family relations.

Not surprisingly, three of the six married women caring for a parent said that they did not want their own children to do the same for them. Mrs Evans saw nothing natural at all about what she was doing and explained her behaviour in terms of the dominant ideology about the role of daughters at the time her mother brought her up (see page 96). She thought that the next generation had adopted new norms of behaviour and that her own children had also been brought up differently by herself:

'I couldn't stand the guilt if we put her in a home and she died. My own children won't feel the same guilt. They've been brought up in an entirely different way. Both my children were clever, and we made up our minds that that was their life.'

Mrs Hall said, 'I've told my children that if I'm running stark naked in a field of snow, leave me there! I know I'd be an old tartar.'

And her words were echoed by Mr and Mrs Archer:

Mr Archer: 'I've told my son to have me put down!'

Mrs Archer: 'All the time you can afford it I'd prefer to pay someone to do it rather than burden the children with it.'

Women caring for a parent-in-law

In this sample there were four women caring for one of their husband's parents: three for a mother-in-law and one for a father-in-law. As was indicated in Chapter 2, these women were the chief carers for their in-laws, and the husbands' contribution to the caring in all but one case was minimal. These relationships were also complicated and difficult; indeed, they included one relationship (Mrs Green) where there was extreme tension between carer and cared for (see page 95 and below). There were strong echoes of the words of those who were caring for their own parents, particularly over questions of power. But there was one new dimension: the carer motivated by maternal and protective feelings for her *husband* – a way of construing the caring relationship to which we return below.

In the section immediately above, we went into some detail about how a number of carers of their mothers claimed that the strength of feeling between themselves and their parents was so strong that either it prevented them from carrying out all caring tasks, or, in order to care properly, they had to ignore or bury those feelings. It is therefore interesting that two of these carers of in-laws claimed that they found it easier to care for their in-laws than they thought it would be to care for one of their own parents. For example, Mrs Davies, who was caring for her father-in-law, said:

'I am emotionally bound up with my mother. Also, she's very irritating, and then I feel guilty. I can't be dispassionate about her, but with my father-in-law I can just shrug it off.'

Later she added, when I asked her if she had any difficulties, 'I can cope. Actually he's very amenable with me. I used to resent it bitterly because he's not a blood relative, though with my mother it would be even more difficult!'

However, despite the fact that Mrs Davies felt she could cope, she did draw the line at the most personal aspects of care. When I asked her what aspect of care she found most difficult, she said:

'Bodily washing him. That's the one problem I didn't feel I could cope with. Now he glorifies in telling me that two nurses at Connors House wash him. I was frightened of his physical strength, and he's much more co-operative with a stranger.'

It is not clear from this quote whether it was feeling – of embarrassment, perhaps – that prevented Mrs Davies from carrying out this particular aspect of very personal care, but it is noteworthy that she herself gave her father-in-law's superior strength as the explanation of her reluctance to bath him. It seems as though the fact that they did *not* share a long and personal history made Mrs Davies's chosen tasks much easier.

Mrs Barnes, who cared for her mother-in-law, also made very similar remarks: 'I don't think I could do it for my own mother, because it would upset me too much.'

Thus these two women tend to confirm my previous argument that when carers refer to the difficulty which 'emotion' or 'feeling' engenders in the caring relationship they are actually saying that the difficulty arises out of the long biography of a relationship and the necessitated change in status from child to quasi-parent and from parent to quasi-child. With in-laws this particular problem of radical change in status is not so acute, since at least the carer and cared for met originally as adults and strangers to each other.

Both these women, despite saying that they would not have been able to care for one of their own parents in the same fashion, nevertheless felt guilty that they were not in a position to offer such care for one of their own parents should it be necessary. For example, Mrs Davies was very anxious about her own 83-year-old mother, who lived many hundreds of miles away and whose paid helper was about to give up:

'I feel very guilty that I'm giving *him* the help she needs. She might have to go into a home if the lady she has to help her now can't manage. Now, there I am much more emotionally involved.'

The thought that her own mother might have to come to live with them and would need the same kind of intensive care that her father-in-law had been receiving from her had created something of a crisis in the Davies household. Mrs Davies felt it quite out of the question that she should care for both elderly people simultaneously; the only way out of the difficulty was if her father-in-law were to enter permanent residential care, but there were considerable problems about this because he was unlikely to be accepted in either the state or the private sector since his

behaviour was very antisocial and disruptive. Much of the interview was taken up with worrying about this problem.

Similarly, but not so acutely, Mrs Barnes felt guilty about
neglecting her own mother:

'I have had very down times because I'm so totally torn. I do
take it quite seriously. I have this ghastly fear of her being found
dead, and then there'd be inquests. It used to play on my mind
terribly; you'd never forgive yourself. I daren't take the risk of
leaving her at night. I used to feel ill, double-locking the door.
But I've felt a bit guilty about my own parents. They're only one
hour away, but I tend to expect them to come here. I often don't
go to them for a year. My mother didn't even tell me about a
recent illness. I thought I'd have to give up Granny if my mother
needed help.'

It does seem that, whoever within their kinship network they
are caring for, women carers feel guilty. One might assume that
women caring for a parent-in-law would not feel as guilty *vis-à-
vis* the rest of their family as women caring for their own parent,
since in caring for a parent-in-law such women are presumably
providing very considerable services to their husbands and, if
there are any, to their husbands' siblings. But clearly this is not
the case. The reason seems to be that, just as with those caring
for their own parents (see pages 127–8), there is a hierarchy of
normative obligations which these women feel they are not
fulfilling. And they are not fulfilling these obligations precisely
because they are spending so much time caring for someone
lower down that normative hierarchy. Paradoxically, by taking
on the care of an in-law, they declare themselves as people who
are motivated by perceived normative obligation and thus make
themselves vulnerable to feelings of guilt about neglecting
someone – their own parent – higher up that hierarchy. In
general, such evidence makes nonsense of broad-brush statements about 'family care' and the need to develop it; 'families'
contain a network of obligations, both nuclear and extended,
and most women seem to have those obligations arranged in
some kind of conceptual hierarchy. Caring, which necessarily
involves very large amounts of time and emotional investment,
almost inevitably involves the transgression of some part of that
network of obligations, whether to children and husband or
to others in the extended kin network. Only women carers,

entirely on their own and without other 'dependants', are likely to be free of guilt.

Mrs Barnes and Mrs Davies also had one other thing in common. Both of them, in slightly different ways and for somewhat different reasons, were very protective of their husbands and took steps to see that their husbands were not upset by the state of their own parents. In certain respects it is arguable that they were pursuing a motherhood model of care, not so much in respect of the person they were caring for, but in respect of their husbands. This was particularly clear with the example of Mrs Davies. Her father-in-law, who did not share the Davies household but lived on his own immediately opposite them, had a long history of mental illness and was now beginning to develop senile dementia. There had been long-standing problems between father and son, which seem to have been exacerbated by the older Mr Davies's developing dependency:

'My husband is an only child. He gets the brunt of his father's aggression. He's the one who tries to exert a little discipline. I've tried to take the load off my husband basically. I began to think my husband was going to get ill; it was to preserve my family that I took over.'

Mrs Davies thus felt that caring for her father-in-law was a means to the further end of caring for her own immediate family, particularly her husband. When I asked her what gave her the most satisfaction about caring, she said, 'It keeps life peaceful for the rest of the family'. At the time of the interview Mrs Davies had persuaded her husband to do less for his father than he had done at one time, because she felt it upset her husband too much.

Mrs Barnes also protected her husband (as well as her brother-in-law and stepson) from seeing the state of her severely senile mother-in-law. This was possible because their mother did not share their immediate household but lived in another house on their small estate about thirty yards from their front door. In this case there was also something of an effort to preserve the old lady's dignity:

'My husband and his brother find it very difficult to cope with. She was always quite happy to be kept in her place by a domineering husband. She's always very cautious about men, and the thought of my husband taking her to the loo is just awful. I try and protect her from that kind of thing. He *does* visit her. She used to come in here all the time. He *has* been up to the hospital with me. . . .

'My husband's been once to see her since she went to the general hospital. I don't think I'd want him to see her in the mental hospital. [Mrs B.'s mother-in-law was, at the time of the interview, temporarily in the local mental hospital for assessment.] . . .

'They won't come to the Carers' Group. They're not medically orientated at all and they can't face it. . . .

'The children didn't see her for a long time. They couldn't cope with it, really. But my daughters are ever so good with her. I can't expect them to do anything for her, though they will if I ask. I wouldn't ask my stepson, and he keeps away. I suppose, again, I've sort of sheltered them. I wouldn't like him to see his grandmother now. He was much closer to her than my daughters. . . .

'In the evenings my daughters used to look in on her every hour, but now she's in such a state that I've stopped them from going in.'

Her mother-in-law left faeces in very odd places:

'That's the worst part of it all. Window-sills are a favourite. It's even been in the fridge! That's really been a big problem – a very big problem. That's really why I've tried to shelter her from other people. It's terribly degrading for her.'

Thus both Mrs Davies and Mrs Barnes apparently saw themselves as the managers of the emotional lives of their families. It was an important part of their role as wives and mothers to ensure the safety and security of *all* the family members; and if that meant that they alone had to shoulder the entire task of caring for the most troubled and troubling member of that family, and keep that person away from the rest of the family – even his or her nearest male relative – then so be it. In this protective mode, I would suggest that a woman carer's motivation can be construed as pursuing the motherhood model of caring for her more immediate family and, in particular, for her husband.

The other two carers of parents-in-law also had something in common. Both of them had problems with their mother-in-law along the dimension of power. Mrs Jackson, whose 92-year-old

mother-in-law had had a stroke and consequently lost her
power of speech but not her facility to communicate volubly
through pencil and paper, felt her mother-in-law as a very
powerful presence within the household. When I asked her
if she experienced any difficulties about caring, Mrs Jackson
replied:

'She's a very strong personality, so she's the one that calls the
tune.'

'For example?'

'Packing for her to go away – she's incredibly particular about
where everything goes.'

'Other difficulties?'

'I'm never at ease with her. I like and admire her, but she
loves arguing about politics, and I don't like arguing at all. I
can't satisfy that need in her at all. She watches telly. We've got
her some headphones because she used to have it on full blast
so that she could hear it. The cooking gets me down; it's such
little messes all the time. I haven't the energy to do separate
meals, so we all eat mashed potato and jelly.'

These problems between the two women had not spilled over
into personal care, which Mrs Jackson was quite happy to do.
The difficulties cropped up in rather less obvious areas. When I
asked Mrs Jackson whether there was anything she couldn't do
for her mother-in-law, she said:

'I'm not prepared to sew for her because I know that whatever
I do would be wrong. We would argue about what was right.'

The worst problems over power seem to have arisen between
Mrs Jackson's teenage children and their grandmother:

'I'm very much aware of the conflict between her and my
children. There's always going to be rows about which television programme to watch and so on.'

'Who wins?'

'She usually does!'

'My daughter and mother-in-law are on the worst terms with
each other. My daughter is really alarmed by her grandmother –
it's the embarrassment over communication. My daughter
resents the whole set-up, really; she's not getting enough
attention. . . .

'The children have already said they will *not* care for us. That's
largely because of having their grandmother. They're completely

irreverent in speaking about her death, in a semi-humorous way. It's had a definite effect on them and made them very much against caring.'

Although there clearly were problems about power in the Jackson household, particularly (though probably not significantly) between the three generations of women in the house, these were as nothing compared to the difficulties that seemed to prevail in the Green household. Mrs Jackson and her mother-in-law at least shared the common ground that the older Mrs Jackson was in need of care and the younger Mrs Jackson was chiefly responsible for providing that care. In contrast, the two Mrs Greens had not as yet reached any kind of equilibrium in their relationship and were not in any agreement as to their respective status as cared for and carer. Mrs Green's mother-in-law had only recently come to live with the Greens, after the death of her husband, Mr Green's father. The main problem seemed to be that Mrs Green thought there was nothing physically wrong with her mother-in-law (see page 95) and considered her to be as able-bodied and as capable of looking after herself and the household as Mrs Green herself was:

'She used to look after father and go up the street every week to get her pension. She used to read five books a week, but she won't read them here! I felt so sorry for her at the beginning I was playing cards with her till midnight. I've broken that now.'

'What parts about caring are most difficult?'

'The daytime, really. You've got to keep an eye on her. She used to moan and groan and say she couldn't be left on her own. But Social Services said she was perfectly capable of being on her own. It's all "me, me, me". It's almost as though *I'm* living with *her*. She won't leave me alone if I'm poorly. She's made me one cup of coffee since she's been here. She won't do anything. . . .

'One part of me says, "Poor old thing". The other part of me says, "Am I living with you or are you living with me?" . . .

'You try so hard. I bought her some slippers; she doesn't like them so she wears my old ones. All my life I've been passing things on to her. . . .

'All her life she used to cook. I gave her brown bread – she threw it at me! She's very choosy. She eats all right now; she used to eat $\frac{1}{2}$ lb of chocolates and three bags of Maltesers a day.

So, as she's had occasional bouts of being runny, I've had to ration her. It's worse than having a child. It doesn't seem right that you should have to do that. . . .

'My husband gets so annoyed, it's unbelievable. He ignores her. But there are awful rows between her and me. He tells me off for listening to her!'

Apparently, then, Mrs Green and her mother-in-law were engaged in something little short of gladiatorial combat. The younger Mrs Green felt sorry for her mother-in-law, not because she was physically incapacitated but because she was recently bereaved. But even in this respect her mother-in-law had let her down:

'She didn't go to Dad's funeral. She just didn't want to know. All she was interested in was getting a widow's pension.'

Mr Green had adopted the strategy of simply withdrawing from the arena:

'Does your husband help?'

'There's a difference between me and him, obviously. He just doesn't take any notice of her, whereas I'm inclined to worry about her.'

It seems to me that most of Mrs Green's problem sprang from the fact that she had not perceived herself to be initiating a caring relationship when her mother-in-law first came to live with them. Given Mrs Green's assumption that there was nothing wrong with her mother-in-law, it followed that she had expected her mother-in-law to provide her with companionship – in other words, that they would be two fully competent women who happened to live in the same house, and who would help each other with the housework and go out and about together:

'My husband says I was silly to think she would change. I thought she would come out with me on outings.'

When I asked Mrs Green whether her mother-in-law gave her anything, such as company, she said very bitterly:

'She's not company; she's asleep, isn't she? That's why I feel she'd be better off with somebody her own age. But then she says, "I'm all right here. You don't want to get rid of me, do you?" And then we have tears. I feel like leaving home for a month and seeing what would happen then.'

The issue about power really devolved into an issue about

dependency, and which of the two women's views as to whether the older Mrs Green needed care or not would prevail. To return to the main theme of Chapter 3, the older Mrs Green seemed to be trying to negotiate her daughter-in-law into the role of carer; as long as the younger Mrs Green refused to accept that role, their battle of wills would continue. At the time of the interview the younger Mrs Green was uncertain how long she could safely leave her mother-in-law alone in the house. Much of the interview was taken up with her worrying away at this question and, in particular, whether she could go on an all-day outing with her husband the following Saturday:

'One part of me says, "You should go out and leave her"; the other part of me says, "Oh, how wicked."'

Mrs Green herself had a bleak view of what the end-result would be if she came to accept her mother-in-law's opinion that she should become a full-time carer:

'At the moment it makes me feel as though I'm never going to get back to what I was. I shall try to get her in permanently for Connors House. If I once get in the habit where I'm staying in all the time, I'll never get out.'

The irony is that, if it really was true that there was nothing wrong with the older Mrs Green, there was no possibility whatever that she would be accepted for permanent care in the recently opened, very high quality, very popular, and very small local-authority unit for residential care. Apparently, Mrs Green had twice previously found warden-assisted flats for her parents-in-law in Canterbury, but each time they had turned the flat down. She had very little hope of persuading her mother-in-law to move into one now, even if such a flat were available. The outlook for this relationship seemed pretty hopeless; each woman had apparently come to it with contradictory expectations. The older Mrs Green (aged 83) seems to have decided that now that her husband was dead she had no one depending on her any more, and it was her right now to extract something from someone else in return; while the younger Mrs Green had hoped that another woman in the house would provide her with the companionship that she wanted, given that before the arrival of her mother-in-law she had been rather lonely. She had wanted to care *about* her mother-in-law rather than care *for* her. Her mother-in-law had wanted precisely the reverse.

THE FUTURE

As must be obvious by now, a number of the carers interviewed in this small study were rather sorry that they had become carers. One out of the four men carers and five out of the fifteen women carers made some kind of statement indicating that they would really strongly prefer some other occupation. Most often these statements were made in answer to a question I asked them about their own future and how they themselves would prefer to be cared for if and when the time came. A number of respondents, including people whom I have not included among those counted as 'unhappy' carers, said something very like the following from Mrs Davies:

'I've told them to take us out and shoot us! They've seen the problems, and we hope we'd have enough sense to put ourselves into a home.'

Very similarly phrased requests for a quite unrealistic form of euthanasia came from Mr and Mrs Archer (see page 129), Mrs Hall (page 129), and Mrs Evans (page 124). Given the references to 'shooting' or, in the case of Mrs Hall, using the traditional Eskimo method of killing off the elderly, I have to assume that these requests were symptomatic and symbolic rather than serious. They indicate a deep unhappiness about informal care. Mrs Evans, Mrs Archer, and Mrs Jackson believed strongly that informal care would have to be replaced by formal care; all three felt that caring should be paid for and never devolve upon a single person as it had done on them. Mrs Evans thought that much more NHS money would have to be spent on caring for the people whom medical technology had kept alive:

'I don't think it's fair. The NHS keeps people alive longer but has not provided the facilities for it; it's a national tragedy.'

Mrs Jackson, like Mrs Archer (see page 129), thought that caring should be paid for and that no individual person should be asked to do it entirely unsupported:

'It immediately puts it all right, doesn't it, if it's somebody's job to do it. And if it's a job, there's a time limit. When she comes back to us [after a few weeks staying with her nieces] it's for ever.'

In contrast, Mrs Barnes, Mrs Cook, and Mrs Lee were confident and expected that their children would care for them. In other words, the problems they were experiencing were not enough, in their opinion, either for them to positively discourage their children from becoming carers, or for their children, having seen the difficulties, simply to opt out. However, as I listened to many of these carers I did come to wonder in what way many of them would eventually be cared for. Those who had adult children found it difficult to see them because they were tied to their own home, and many had great difficulty making time to see friends and neighbours. They were thus in danger of losing kin and neighbourhood networks that *might*, if the need ever arose, provide the same kind of care that they were providing for their elderly relative. The prospect for many of them really did seem rather grim, only alleviated for some by the possibility of paying for their own care in East Kent's mushrooming private care system. But there is little doubt that caring itself had depressed their incomes over their working lifetimes, so that one has to presume that, unless eligible for full DHSS funding via the Social Fund (Bradshaw 1987), many, if not most, would be unable to purchase their own care in the private sector. A shrinking and stigmatized public sector or a very lonely old age, with rather sporadic Social Services support, seemed to be the prospect for many of these fully committed informal carers. As Mrs Evans said, in another context, 'It isn't fair.'

7
Conclusions: morality, identity, and public responsibility

It is not easy to bring this book to an end. In my view there cannot and should not be an 'end' in the sense of a satisfactory conclusion to the narrative. The exploratory nature of the original research proposals, the open-endedness of the interviews, the lack of clear policy-oriented focus, and the complexity of the issues raised in the course of the interviews with carers all mean that I cannot finish neatly, either with a firm assertion of a hypothesis proved or disproved, or with the clear set of prescriptive suggestions with which books on social-policy-related topics often, and quite rightly, close. This has been a different kind of book. I have tried to describe, at a material and ideological level, the reasons why the particular men and women in my sample came to be 'carers' and how they made sense of their position. The answers they themselves gave me and the motivations I have ascribed to them are not cut and dried; they are complicated, often in self-contradiction and hence full of tension, sometimes apparently highly personal and yet, I have claimed, generalizable. It is for others to decide whether these generalizations are legitimate or useful; it is my hope that they will constitute the tools for further – perhaps deeper and more broadly based – interdisciplinary research and speculation.

Meantime, however, it is possible to extract some strands from this narrative with which to draw to an end. Throughout the book I have stressed the material and ideological determinants of the decision to care. But throughout the interviews I was aware that what people were describing to me was their own beliefs about 'right' and 'wrong' and their personal struggles to enact their moral beliefs and sort out their moral dilemmas. While these beliefs can be called 'ideology' (and loosely this is what I have meant by the phrase), this term is far too over-arching and deterministic to capture the complexity of the essentially moral decisions that these carers regularly made in their daily lives. Without exception, all of them felt that gendered kinship formed the basis for a general system of morality. But within that general system, there were variations between carers as to hierarchies of obligation, disagreements among them as to how far others, particularly their own children, should be similarly obligated, expectations among many of them that the nature of 'good' behaviour could and would alter over the generations, and an understanding that the quantity and quality of state intervention in provision for dependent people was a major determinant of the basis for private morality. While the carers themselves were moral agents, constantly working out a moral stance on particular issues, many of them also understood that they were acted *upon*, even to the extent of being moral *victims*.

It seems that moral rules have a peculiar longevity, despite the claims by those on the political right that the public morality of the Welfare State has recently reduced us as individuals to the status of amoral sponges. But it would be a mistake to think that every one of us is driven by the same concepts of 'duty' or 'love' as the carers in this sample. During the interviews I have frequently become acutely aware of 'absent friends'. The shadowy figures of alternative carers have featured in almost all these conversations, but none of these alternative carers, for one reason or another, has ever seemed the 'right' person to care for the particular dependent adult in question (see Chapter 3). Only on rare occasions have the carers in this sample indicated resentment about the lack of support, practical and moral, received from other members of their kin network.

In other words, in this study I have looked at the people who, when faced with a particular constellation of moral problems, have followed their understanding of the imperatives of gendered kinship and the obligations of marriage 'in sickness and in health'. At the same time, I have been aware that there are others in many of these carers' networks who have followed a different path and, implicitly or explicitly, have said 'no'. It would be wrong to assume that these people who have said 'no' are in some sense immoral, less 'good', and more prepared to depend on the provisions of the state than the people who have said 'yes'. As the discussion in Chapter 6 shows, many of the carers interviewed here felt that not only had *they* made sacrifices, but so, willy-nilly, had other members of their family networks, including other elderly frail relatives for whom they were not caring, and their own husbands and children. As was indicated in Chapter 3, almost all the carers interviewed in this study thought that, where there did seem to be potential alternative carers in their gendered kin networks, these alternative carers had had legitimate reasons for saying 'no'. From this one can infer one of two possibilities: first, that among those who have said 'no' are those who are operating a very slightly different set of moral imperatives, where other members of the gendered kinship and marriage network are regarded as making higher and stronger claims on the nurturing services and emotional management of an alternative potential carer. The fact that most of the carers in this sample thought that the process by which they had become carers was in some sense 'obvious' indicated that, however hard the consequences for them personally, they accepted and agreed with the alternative moral imperatives under which the potential alternative carers were operating.

However, it might equally be possible that those who said 'no' simply had more power within their family networks to be effectively negative; in other words, in a postulated battle to avoid gendered kinship obligations the eventual carer was the one who 'lost'. Carers have until recently been invisible, but now I think there is an even more invisible group whom we need to know more about: the 'non-carers'. Who are these non-carers and what determines their strength to say 'no'? Why do their families accept their reasons for not caring as legitimate? These are not just interesting questions with a largely sociological import; there are also good social policy reasons for asking them. We are increasingly moving to a situation where – to borrow a term from the professional world of community care – it is the informal carers who are going to be the 'case managers' chiefly responsible for the organization and procurement of the appropriate care 'package' for the person they are caring for. From the data presented here it is evident that gender and the nature of the kin relationship between carer and cared for are the dominant determining factors in selecting the carer; but some carers also suggested that there were other important considerations in selecting out a possible alternative carer, particularly perceptions about the relative importance of careers (either the non-carer's or her husband's). If the careers and articulated reluctance of the alternative carers are also significant determining factors in the selection of a carer, then it might well be that those who became carers are the least well-off and, possibly, the least assertive members of a family network. This may have implications for the quality of care that they can procure.

During this research I have been struck by two quite different kinds of carer, particularly among the women: those for whom caring was truly grim, and those for whom it seemed to bestow a certain satisfaction, even, in one or two cases, an extraordinary kind of joy. I could not make sense of this at all, except, in the case of the joyful carers, to think, generously, in terms of genuine saintliness, or less sanguinely and much more arrogantly, in terms of false consciousness. Only recently, on happening upon a story about George Eliot – who from age 16 to 30 cared for her own father – did the picture begin to clarify. In her middle age Eliot was a frequent visitor to Cambridge. Frederic Myers, a Fellow of Trinity College, recalled a visit by her in 1873:

'She, stirred somewhat beyond her wont, and taking as her text the three words that have been used so often as the inspiring trumpet-calls of men – the words, God, Immortality, Duty – pronounced, with terrible earnestness, how inconceivable was the first, how unbelievable the second, and yet how peremptory and absolute the third. Never, perhaps, have sterner accents affirmed the sovereignty of impersonal and unrecompensating Law. I listened and night fell; her grave, majestic countenance turned towards me like a sibyl's in the gloom; it was as though she withdrew from my grasp, one by one, the two scrolls of promise, and left me the third scroll only, awful with inevitable fates. And when we stood at length and parted, amid that columnar circuit of forest-trees, beneath the last twilight of starless skies, I seemed to be gazing, like Titus at Jerusalem, on vacant seats and empty halls – on a sanctuary with no Presence to hallow it, and heaven left lonely of a God.'

(cited in Haight 1968)

(Apparently, Bertrand Russell in his *Autobiography* recalled the story in rather less stentorian tones. He was told: 'This is where George Eliot told F. W. H. Myers that there is no God and yet we must be good; and Myers decided there is a God and yet we need not be good.')

It is precisely that grim call of 'duty' to which George Eliot referred in the gloom which so many of the women carers in this sample felt they were trapped by. For most of these carers, the 'vacant seats and empty halls' were not only unhallowed by a 'Presence', they were also, rather more prosaically, unoccupied by many (or any?) people who could observe and approve of what they were doing. These carers were, indeed, the 'forgotten army' (Henwood and Wicks 1984), unmentioned in dispatches by a government which assumed, if they were female, that they were at home anyway (Groves and Finch 1983), and frequently cut off from possible observation and approval by their wider family, friends, and neighbours. Their one comfort might be that the 'vacant seats and empty halls' are now beginning to fill a little; the movement of the term 'carer' into the vernacular, the arrival of Carers' Support Groups, and the growth of research and publication in the area of caring have all helped a small amount to alleviate 'duty' with 'recognition' if not with 'reward'. (Even 'reward' has been added to in a small way very recently, with the success of the test claim for the Invalid Care Allowance brought by Mrs Jacqueline Drake to the European Court of Justice.)

But what of the 'joyful' carers? There were not many of these, it must be said, but they included a handful of women and, stretching the point somewhat, three of the men. 'Joy' is perhaps an exaggerated term to use; what I mean is a general air of considerable contentment in circumstances which many others would, and do, find distressing, depressing, and disturbing.

One basis for explaining both the contented women carers (as well as the fact that at least two of them seemed to have sought out people to care for) and the attitudes of the men carers might lie in the book by Carol Gilligan, *In a Different Voice* (1982). Gilligan, a psychologist, argues that as a result of boys' and girls' differential Oedipal development little girls and boys form their feminine and masculine identity differently:

> 'relationships, and particularly issues of dependency, are experienced differently by men and women. For boys and men, separation and individuation are critically tied to gender identity since separation from the mother is essential for the development of masculinity. For girls and women, issues of femininity or feminine identity do not depend on the achievement of separation from the mother or on the progress of individuation. Since masculinity is defined through separation while femininity is defined through attachment, male gender identity is threatened by intimacy while female gender identity is threatened by separation. Thus males tend to have difficulty with relationships, while females tend to have problems with individuation.'

> (Gilligan 1982: 8)

Gilligan asserts that the end-result of these differential Oedipal experiences of infant boys and girls is that mature men and women have different moral frameworks and ways of approaching moral questions. Men refer to rights, which are subject to public and rational assessment; women refer to responsibilities, which are private and sensitive to individuals and their particular relationships:

> 'Women's deference is rooted not only in their social subordination but also in the substance of their moral concern. Sensitivity to the needs of others and the assumption of responsibility for taking care lead women to attend to voices other than their own and to include in their judgment other points of view. Women's moral weakness, manifest in an apparent diffusion and confusion of judgment, is thus inseparable from women's moral strength, an overriding concern with relationships and responsibilities. The reluctance to judge may itself be indicative of the care and concern for

others that infuse the psychology of women's development and are responsible for what is generally seen as problematic in its nature. *Thus women not only define themselves in a context of human relationships but also judge themselves in terms of their ability to care.* Women's place in man's life cycle has been that of nurturer, caretaker, and helpmate, the weaver of those networks of relationships on which she in turn relies.'

(1982: 16–17; my italics)

Within this analysis by Gilligan, it might be possible to explain these apparently 'joyful' carers – at least as far as the women are concerned. She would presumably suggest that the 'contented' women carers in this study were those who felt that through caring they were making and fulfilling their *female* identity. She would suggest that the origins of their need to express their female identity by fulfilling the needs of others lie deep in their childhood development; their success at caring for others meant they judged themselves with a light touch.

This, of course, does not explain the grim commitment to 'duty' that so many of the other women carers claimed to be their motivation and which so many regretted. For them, the calls of 'duty' and the way that concept particularly applies to women are clearly less to do with the expression of sex *differences* and female identity and more to do with the expectations of society at large of sex *roles*. Far from understanding their motivation in terms of a claim to an essentially feminine identity, these 'dutiful' women carers seemed to feel that their very and visible femaleness had placed them in an especially vulnerable position *vis-à-vis* the demands of the state, their families and the perceived needs of the dependent person in their immediate kin network.

These different explanations of the motivation of women to care – the one essentially conservative, rooted in childhood and explained by psychology; the other essentially dynamic, rooted in society and explained by sociology – have, in the British literature on caring, been brought together by Hilary Graham in an essay entitled 'Caring: A Labour of Love' (1983). (Although Graham's work was published in 1983 it was written well before Gilligan's work was generally available in the UK. Graham referred to the work of feminist psychologist Nancy Chodorow

(1978) in much the same way as Gilligan.) In her essay, Graham argues that psychologists and social policy analysts are essentially addressing different aspects of caring. Psychologists look to its affective components and its peculiar affinity with femininity, while social policy analysts look to the function of family care within capitalism and patriarchy. In so doing both disciplines make fundamental errors:

> 'The psychological studies tell us what caring means in emotional terms, but not in material terms. By neglecting the material basis of caring, an aspect so central to the understanding of gender relations, the psychological perspective is seen to run dangerously close to essentialism, to an argument that caring reflects women's biological nature and women's psychic needs. . . . The more recent work within social policy, particularly that initiated by marxist-feminist writers, has corrected this tendency by focusing on caring (and dependency) as a political and economic relation supported by the wider system of gender divisions. In spelling out the material benefits for the state, this work has highlighted the exploitation of women's labour on which the present organisation of family care rests. In so doing it tends to underplay the symbolic bonds that hold the caring relationship together. The roots of people's deep resistance to the socialisation of care is thus lost. Whether provided through the institutions of the state or through the intervention of "good neighbours" in the community, both carers and their dependants recognise that the substitute services are not "care", since they lack the very qualities of commitment and affection which transform caring-work into a life-work, a job into a duty.'
>
> (Graham 1983: 28–9)

Graham concludes that the two ways of thinking about caring can be brought together through the development of an understanding

> 'that caring defines *both* the identity *and* the activity of women in Western society. It defines what it feels like to be a woman in a male-dominated and capitalist social order. Men negotiate their social position through something recognised as "doing", "doing" based on "knowledge" which enables them to "think"

and engage in "skilled work". Women's social position is negotiated through a different kind of activity called "caring", a caring informed not by knowledge but by "intuition" through which women find their way into "unskilled" jobs.

(1983: 30)

Graham's attempt at bridge-building between psychology and social policy analysis seems to me to be wholly laudable (and this book is perhaps an empirical example of a similar attempt to build bridges between these two disciplines). However, it is perhaps not surprising to find, even in the small sample of carers discussed here, possible examples – on the one hand – of women carers who have found their female identity through caring, and yet – on the other – of others who feel exploited and who bitterly regret their loss of autonomy and identity because, through the operation of gendered expectations and obligations, their own needs have had to become subordinate to the more pressing needs of someone else. In other words, it may be the case that Chodorow and Gilligan's kind of psychological analysis can exhaustively explain the 'voluntary' motivation of *some* female carers, while more material sociological analysis of women's position under capitalism, and social policy analysis of the state's assumption of the availability of women for caring, can more properly explain the 'enforced' motivation of *other* female carers. Conceptual bridge-building of the Graham kind may not reflect a dichotomized reality.

It is also useful to consider Gilligan's (1982) analysis and its applicability to understanding the motivation of the men carers. As was outlined in Chapter 4, the four men carers were all caring for their wives, and three of them spoke of their motivation in terms of 'love'. Most of the women, in contrast, spoke of their motivation in terms of 'duty'. At first sight this seems incompatible with Gilligan's view that it is women, rather than men, who base their moral judgements on responsibilities arising from relationships, while men base their judgements on questions of rights. However, it seems to me at least arguable that the term 'love' was being used by the men as shorthand to indicate the constellation of rights and obligations contained in the marriage vows and to which they had committed themselves, on marriage, for life. The use of the word 'love' might also be said to have two further qualities; it is less grim and more comfortable than 'duty' and it is also far more active. In this context, then, it seems that Graham's essay (1983) is just as relevant to the findings in this study. As she points out (in words already quoted on page 148): 'Men negotiate their social position through something recognised as "doing", "doing", based on "knowledge" which enables them to "think" and engage in "skilled work"' (1983: 30). In the discussion of how three of the four men carers talked about the process of caring (see Chapter 6) it was argued that they used occupational language drawn from the labour market to describe the work; two of them also clearly understood that, through the experience of caring, they had acquired a set of transferable skills. This was in marked contrast to almost all the women carers, for whom the skills of caring appeared to come 'automatically'.

To return to the more material matters with which this study originated (see Chapter 1), the initiating question concerned the impact of women's participation in the labour market on the 'caring capacity of the community'. In an earlier piece of work I argued that it was doubtful if the growth of women's paid work, particularly in part-time employment, would have any great impact on the eventual availability of individual women to care (Ungerson 1981, 1983a). There is nothing in this study to contradict that previous view, although a study of 'non-carers' might reveal something. However, it seems to me that there is another material change that has taken place recently and will continue to have a cross-generational impact on caring for many years to come. This is the very rapid recent increase in owner-occupation, from 29 per cent of the dwelling stock in the UK in 1951 to 61 per cent in 1984 (CSO 1986). As a result, over the next thirty or forty years very large numbers of people and households will accrue over their lifetimes a considerable amount of capital in the form of property. Towards the end of their lives, if the housing market behaviour of elderly owner-occupiers remains much the same as it is at present, old people are likely to capitalize some or all of this property and either move down-market or take out some form of annuity based on the value of their property. This does not seem to me to have an immediate gendered implication. Yet it reminds us that families are not just the loci for relationships based on affection, history, and gendered obligations. Families are also the locus of relationships based on *property relations*, and will increasingly be so.

At the same time as some old people are acquiring substantial amounts of capital, there are very rapid developments taking place in the field of private-sector systems of community care. Examples are the rapid growth in private sheltered housing, the mushrooming of private residential and nursing-homes, particularly on the South Coast (Audit Commission 1986) and most visibly in the one-time popular holiday resorts of East Kent, the development of private or full-cost alarm systems, and private home-help and nursing services. Thus in some households (perhaps even the majority), particularly those where substantial gains have been made through owner-occupation, it will be possible to avoid some or all of the tasks of informal care through the purchase of private-sector systems of care. This will happen, however, only at huge cost to the old people themselves and/or to their families. According to the Audit Commission (1986), the costs of care for a frail elderly person in a private-sector residential home were £138.55 per week at 1986 prices, and in a private nursing-home were £183.55.

Given that private systems of care are growing, and increasing numbers of old people, through moving downmarket in the owner-occupied sector, are going to be able to afford to pay the very high costs that prevail in that sector, we need to bear in mind two points. First, there are limits to the expansion of owner-occupation, and there will remain within the foreseeable future a substantial minority of the population who will not have access to this method of subsidized capital accumulation. This will give rise to general social divisions and differences and will also exacerbate existing social divisions in the ability of families to generate support services for their carers. Propertied carers will have to fend off the blandishments of ever increasing numbers of private operators in this field, while the non-propertied carers will be increasingly dependent on state services whose future is uncertain, to say the least. Secondly, and related to this point, even among those who have succeeded in accumulating large amounts of capital over their lifetimes, there will be considerable differences – often depending on arbitrary factors such as whether they had the good fortune to live in Aberdeen in the 1960s and 1970s or London in the 1980s. The result of these differences, between those with large amounts of property and those with none or considerably less, is that it is inevitable, if the public sector of care fails to keep up with demand, that an extremely stratified system of care will emerge.

Some households (containing many Conservative voters who would normally support 'family' based policies?) will be able to demonstrate that informal care is not necessarily what many people prefer, by voting with their feet for the alternative of private residential care. (However, it is ironic that they may not be able to use their feet, and large amounts of money, to generate very high-quality care. Despite the Registered Homes Act 1984, the difficulties entailed in ongoing regulation of the private sector may mean that these households could find themselves in receipt of private services that lack provision for 'privacy, dignity, autonomy and individuality' in precisely the same way as the heavily criticized institutional public-sector care (Vyvyan 1987). It is also ironic that it was such criticism of public-sector residential care, particularly in the large mental hospitals, which in the 1960s laid the moral basis for the initial political consensus in favour of community care and its continuing support from the present Conservative government – see Chapter 1.) Meanwhile, those dependent on the public sector for support services for informal carers, and/or the permanent alternative of state-funded residential care, will find themselves as ill-supported, isolated and depressed as many of the carers, particularly the poorer ones, described in the pages of this book. As the robust and anonymous authors of the Audit Commission report put it:

'If nothing changes, the outlook is bleak. Community care policies are being adopted to a limited degree only, with slow and uneven progress across the country. For mentally ill and elderly people the following trends are evident:

(a) Long-stay hospital provision is being reduced at a significant rate, on a pro-rata basis for elderly people and absolutely for the mentally ill.

(b) But local authority community-based services are not expanding sufficiently rapidly to offset the rundown in NHS accommodation; and no one knows what has happened to many of the patients that have been discharged.

(c) Provision of community-based local authority support services is very uneven; in some areas it is close to non-existent for mentally ill people in particular.'

(Audit Commission 1986: 26)

In my view it would be a disgrace and a tragedy if we allowed a hugely stratified system of care for the elderly to develop in the UK. This book has described how the responsibility for informal care is at present stratified by sex; the introduction of further stratification, largely determined by social and housing class position, would make the informal care system even more unfair than it already is. If, through the neglect of a properly funded system of public-sector support services for carers and a failure to provide high-quality publicly funded and accountable residential care for the frail, we encourage a major development of private-sector care, we will not only be introducing a very important new form of social division within British society as a whole; we will also be encouraging the development of acute divisions within families. For, given the prices charged for residential care and support services within the private and profit-making sector, there is little or no doubt that, if there is an 'obvious' woman carer within a kin network, then enormous and concerted pressure will be brought to bear on her by her own kin in order to help preserve the eventual family inheritance. On every count, then, the neglect of properly funded public and universalist community-care services is a thoroughly divisive policy. It will set rich against poor, brother against sister.

Unless the reality of community care becomes something considerably more than is currently promised, let alone planned for, it is difficult to see how it can possibly remain a politically popular policy. The great swing in public sentiment against care for people in residential institutions that has characterized the last thirty years is, in my opinion, faltering and doing so for the very good reason that community care, as presently constituted, is rapidly coming to be understood as essentially cost-cutting rather than liberalizing and liberating. This is a true 'women's issue'; it cuts across class and political-party allegiance. Every woman in the UK, of whatever social class and income position, who is in touch with living parents or parents-in-law, faces the problem of and responsibility for their care at some point in her life. That this is so, and is generally understood as such, is supported by evidence from a team of researchers who in the early 1980s carried out a large-scale survey of attitudes to informal and formal care in three urban areas in Scotland. In order to ascertain what people thought about different forms of care, the researchers presented their random sample with 'vignettes' describing the position of six kinds of dependent people and asked their respondents to select a preferred form of care among a list of options – ranging from family care only to full-time and permanent residential care. As far as care for the elderly was concerned, the large majority (58 per cent) went for sheltered housing as the most appropriate form of care for the physically handicapped elderly, while an even larger majority (66 per cent) preferred permanent residential care in an old people's home or a geriatric hospital for a confused elderly person. In both cases, very low proportions thought family care only was an appropriate form of care, and overwhelming numbers of women in particular rejected informal care, and even informal care with domiciliary professional help, for the confused elderly (West, Illsley, and Kelman 1984). Indeed, the one variable that appeared to make any significant difference to the replies of the people surveyed was their sex; women, irrespective of their past voting patterns, their social class, and whether or not they had 'traditional' views about family life, were even less in favour of family care only than were men, and were the more likely to prefer care solutions that involved a great deal of professional and Social Service input (West *et al*, 1984).

Such findings indicate that large majorities of the British population are sensitively aware of the kind of problem to which informal care, totally without or only minimally supported by the professional Social Services, can give rise. It is ironic and paradoxical that the alternative to care organized and provided by that most hierarchical and task-divided set of professions – namely, health-care personnel – should be devolving on to the single carer working alone in her own home carrying out, all day and every day, all the tasks akin to those of the nurse, the home help, the care assistant, and the 'social care manager'. In the short run, and even in the long run, I doubt if we can realistically expect there to be a radical shift of the sexual division of labour in both the public and private domains, such that men, irrespective of their position in the life cycle, will be prevailed upon to be 'available' as informal carers in the same way as women are at present. In other words, we have to find public ways of supporting carers that recognize that women, who predominate among carers, are at present being unfairly and unreasonably exploited and that they should have substantial support which takes account of their particular needs. I would argue that the answer is not cash benefits or 'wages for caring' (Fairbairns 1979) payable directly to carers for the work that they do (although under certain circumstances that would be a help), since, given that most carers are women, this will serve to lock them further into sole responsibility for caring work, and would constitute a further incentive for women to give up rather more adequately paid work in the labour market in order to take on the full-time care for someone frail and elderly in their kin network. Rather than cash support, what is needed is high-quality and easily available domiciliary and day-care *services*, combined with equally high-quality forms of flexible residential care, including permanent sheltered housing for protected independent living and regular respite care for those normally cared for informally. Such services must be allocated in such a way that they sensitively take account of the problems arising out of intimate care between close kin with a long biography. As this study has shown, informal care between family members is very far from being unproblematic; it can, and almost always does, raise in acute form issues of power, bereavement for the loss of a loved personality, anxiety about sole responsibility, and feelings of exploitation and manipulation. As was argued in Chapter 1, public policy, particularly for community care, has a fundamental impact on personal life; similarly personal life must have an impact on public policy.

References

Audit Commission for Local Authorities in England and Wales (1986) *Making a Reality of Community Care*. London: HMSO.

Baldwin, S. (1985) *The Costs of Caring: Families with Disabled Children*. London: Routledge & Kegan Paul.

Bayley, M. (1973) *Mental Handicap and Community Care*. London: Routledge & Kegan Paul.

Bebbington, A. C. and Davies, B. (1983) Equity and Efficiency in the Allocation of the Personal Social Services. *Journal of Social Policy* 12, pt 3, July: 309–30.

Bradshaw, J. (1987) The Social Fund. In M. Brenton and C. Ungerson (eds) *The Year Book of Social Policy, 1986/87*. London: Longman.

Bulmer, M. (1986) *Neighbours: The Work of Philip Abrams*. Cambridge: Cambridge University Press.

Central Statistical Office (1986) *Social Trends 16, 1986 Edition*. London: HMSO.

Chodorow, N. (1978) *The Reproduction of Mothering*. Berkeley: University of California Press.

Cohen, G. (ed.) (1987) *Social Change and the Life Course*. London: Tavistock.

Cmnd 1604 (1962) *A Hospital Plan for England and Wales*. London: HMSO.

Cmnd 1973 (1963) *Health and Welfare: The Development of Community Care*. London: HMSO.

Equal Opportunities Commission (1980) *The Experience of Caring for Elderly and Handicapped Dependants: Survey Report*. Manchester: EOC.

—— (1982a), *Caring for the Elderly and Handicapped: Community Care Policies and Women's Lives*. Manchester: EOC.

—— (1982b) *Who Cares for the Carers? Opportunities for Those Caring for the Elderly and Handicapped*. Manchester: EOC.

Fairbairns, Z. (1979) The Cohabitation Rule – Why It Makes Sense. *Women's Studies International Quarterly* 2: 319–27.

Finch, J. and Groves, D. (1980) Community Care and the Family: A Case for Equal Opportunities? *Journal of Social Policy* 9, pt 4, October: 487–511.

—— and —— (eds) (1983) *A Labour of Love: Women, Work and Caring*. London; Routledge & Kegan Paul.

Gilligan, C. (1982) *In a Different Voice: Psychological Theory and Women's Development*. Cambridge, Mass., and London: Harvard University Press.

Graham, H. (1983) Caring: A Labour of Love. In Finch and Groves (1983). *op. cit.*

Groves, D. and Finch, J. (1983) Natural Selection: Perspectives on Entitlement to the Invalid Care Allowance. In Finch and Groves (1983).

Haight, G. S. (1968) *George Eliot: A Biography*. Oxford: Clarendon Press.

Health and Welfare: The Development of Community Care (1963). London: HMSO, Cmnd 1973.

Henwood, M. (1986) Community Care: Policy, Practice and Prognosis. In M. Brenton and C. Ungerson (eds) *The Year Book of Social Policy in Britain 1985–86*. London: Routledge & Kegan Paul.

Henwood, M. and Wicks, M. (1984) *The Forgotten Army: Family Care and Elderly People*. London: Family Policy Studies Centre.

Holme, A. (1985) *Housing and Young Families in East London*. London: Routledge & Kegan Paul.

A Hospital Plan for England and Wales (1962). London: HMSO, Cmnd 1604.

Jones, K. and Fowles, A. J. (1984) *Ideas on Institutions: Analysing the Literature of Long-Term Care and Custody*. London: Routledge & Kegan Paul.

Land, H. (1978) Who Cares for the Family? *Journal of Social Policy*, 7, pt 3, July: 257–84.

Levin, E., Sinclair, I., and Gorbach, P. (1983) *The Supporters of Confused Elderly People: Extract from the Main Report*. London: National Institute for Social Work Research Unit.

McIntosh, M. (1979) The Welfare State and the Needs of the Dependent Family. In S. Burman (ed.) *Fit Work for Women*. London: Croom Helm.

Martin, J. and Roberts, C. (1984) *Women and Employment: A Lifetime Perspective*. London: HMSO.

Moroney, R. M. (1976) *The Family and the State: Considerations for Social Policy*. London: Longman.

Nissel, M. and Bonnerjea, L. (1982) *Family Care of the Handicapped Elderly: Who Pays?* London: Policy Studies Institute.

Office of Population, Censuses and Surveys (OPCS) (1984) *The General Household Survey 1983*. London: HMSO.

Pahl, R. E. (1984) *Divisions of Labour*. Oxford: Blackwell.

Parker, G. (1985) *With Due Care and Attention: A Review of Research on Informal Care*. Occasional Paper No. 2. London: Family Policy Studies Centre.

Qureshi, H. and Walker, A. (forthcoming) *The Caring Relationship: The Family Care of Elderly People*.

Renvoize, J. (1982) *Incest: A Family Pattern*. London: Routledge & Kegan Paul.

Roberts, H. (ed.) (1981) *Doing Feminist Research*. London: Routledge & Kegan Paul.

Social Science Research Council (1980) *Research in Social Administration* (circular letter, 28 February).

Stacey, M. (1981) The Division of Labour Revisited or Overcoming the Two Adams. In P. Abrams, R. Deem, J. Finch, and P. Rock (eds) *Practice and Progress: British Sociology 1950–1980*. London: Allen & Unwin.

Titmuss, R. (1968) Community Care: Fact or Fiction? In R. Titmuss, *Commitment to Welfare*. London: Allen & Unwin.

Townsend, P. (1957) *The Family Life of Old People*. London: Routledge & Kegan Paul.

Townsend, P. (1962) *The Last Refuge: A Survey of Residential Institutions and Homes of Old People*. London: Routledge & Kegan Paul.

Ungerson, C. (1981) *Women, Work and the 'Caring Capacity of the Community': A Report of a Research Review*. Report to the SSRC, mimeo.

—— (1983a) Why Do Women Care? In Finch and Groves (1983).

—— (1983b) Women and Caring: Skills, Tasks and Taboos. In E. Gamarnikow, D. Morgan, J. Purvis, and D. Taylorson (eds) *The Public and the Private*. London: Heinemann.

—— (1985a) *Gender Divisions and Community Care*. End-of-award report to the ESRC. (Lodged at British Library Lending Division.)

—— (1985b) Paid Work and Unpaid Caring: A Problem for Women or the State? In P. Close and R. Collins (eds) *Family and Economy in Modern Society*. London: Macmillan.

—— (1987) The Life Course and Informal Caring: Towards a Typology. In G. Cohen (ed.) *Social Change and the Life Course*. London: Tavistock.

Vyvyan, C. (1987) The Registered Homes Act 1984: Reform and

Response. In M. Brenton and C. Ungerson (eds) *The Year Book of Social Policy 1986/7*. London: Longman.

West, P. (1984) The Family, the Welfare State and Community Care: Political Rhetoric and Public Attitudes. *Journal of Social Policy*, 13, pt 4, October: 417–46.

West, P., Illsley, R., and Kelman, H. (1984) Public Preferences for the Care of Dependency Groups. *Social Science and Medicine*, 18, 4: 287–95.

Wilkin, D. (1979) *Caring for the Mentally Handicapped Child*. London: Croom Helm.

Willmott, P. (1986) *Social Networks, Informal Care and Public Policy*. London: Policy Studies Institute.

Wright, F. (1986) *Left to Care Alone*. Aldershot: Gower.

Name index

The names used for respondents in the research sample appear in the subject index.

Subject index